Smoothies Targeted for Specific Health Issues

73 Superfood Smoothie Recipes for 14 Ailments: Alzheimer's, Arthritis, Cancer, Cholesterol, Diabetes, Heart Disease and More

By Karen C Groves

Copyright © 2013 Network Performance Corporation.
ALL RIGHTS RESERVED.

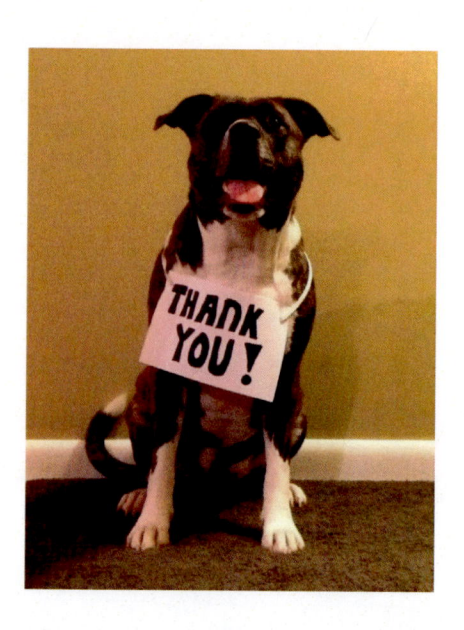

Thank you for downloading our book. Please review it on Amazon so that we can make future versions even better. Thank You So Much!

Get Your Free Supplement

We've published a supplement to this Superfoods Series, *Superfood Fruit Health Benefits*. This supplement is yours **FREE** by writing us at npc_pubs@comcast.net, with your name and best email address, and with 'Superfoods Supplement' in the Subject line. We'll send it to you by return email.

We thrive on constructive criticism from our readers and will acknowledge great comments and suggestions that we use in future editions of these books. Sent them to npc_pubs@comcast.net, with 'Superfoods - Suggestions' in the Subject line. We will add you to an 'Acknowledgements' page when we use your inputs.

NOTE: We respect your privacy and never share your information with anyone.

Table of Contents

WHAT'S THIS BOOK ALL ABOUT? AND WHY? 6
INTRODUCTION 7
MAKING THE SMOOTHIES 10
    Tips and Suggestions 10
    Blenders 12
ALZHEIMER'S AND DEMENTIA 14
    About Alzheimer's and Dementia 14
    Role of Superfoods in Alzheimer's and Dementia 16
    Smoothies for Alzheimer's and Dementia 17
ARTHRITIS / RHEUMATOID ARTHRITIS 19
    About Arthritis / Rheumatoid Arthritis 19
    Role of Superfoods in Arthritis / Rheumatoid Arthritis 21
    Smoothies for Arthritis / Rheumatoid Arthritis 22
ASTHMA 25
    About Asthma 25
    Role of Superfoods in Asthma 27
    Smoothies for Asthma 28
CANCER 30
    About Cancer 30
    Role of Superfoods in Cancer 33
    Smoothies for Cancer 34
CHOLESTEROL 38
    About Cholesterol 38
    Role of Superfoods in Managing Cholesterol 40
    Smoothies for Managing Cholesterol 41
DEPRESSION 43
    About Depression 43
    Role of Superfoods in Depression 45
    Smoothies for Depression 46
DIABETES 48
    About Diabetes 48

Role of Superfoods in Diabetes 50
Smoothies for Diabetes 51

EYESIGHT/ MACULAR DEGENERATION/ BLINDNESS 53
About Eyesight/ Macular Degeneration/ Blindness 53
Role of Superfoods in Eyesight/ Macular Degeneration/
Blindness 55
Smoothies for Eyesight/ Macular Degeneration/ Blindness
.... 56

FIBROMYALGIA 59
About Fibromyalgia 59
Role of Superfoods in Fibromyalgia 61
Smoothies for Fibromyalgia 62

GOUT 64
About Gout 64
Role of Superfoods in Gout 64
Smoothies for Gout 66

HEART DISEASE/ HYPERTENSION/ STROKE 68
About Heart Disease/ Hypertension/ Stroke 68
Role of Superfoods in Heart Disease 71
Smoothies for Heart Health 73

INFLAMMATION 77
About Inflammation 77
Role of Superfoods in Inflammation 79
Smoothies for Inflammation 80

LOW LIBIDO/ ERECTILE DYSFUNCTION 81
About Low Libido/ Erectile Dysfunction 81
Role of Superfoods in Libido/ Erectile Function 83
Smoothies for Libido and Erectile Function and More 84

OSTEOPOROSIS 86
About Osteoporosis 86
Role of Superfoods in Osteoporosis 88
Smoothies for Osteoporosis 89

CONCLUSION 90

RECOMMENDED READS AND RESOURCES 92

APPENDIX I – DISEASE STATISTICS 96

APPENDIX II – OUR HEALTH AND OUR FOOD 99
APPENDIX III - SUPPLEMENTATION 101
APPENDIX IV – SELF MUSCLE TESTING 103
ABOUT THE AUTHOR 105
COPYRIGHT NOTICE AND DISCLAIMER 107

WHAT'S THIS BOOK ALL ABOUT? AND WHY?

I've been working with health issues like cancer and diabetes, and with natural products and supplements for over 20 years, and with superfoods specifically for several years – motivated by the dangerously poor quality of our food supply. And I've been 'playing' with smoothie recipes and drinking smoothies a lot.

So when my publisher asked me to develop and write about smoothies targeted at specific ailments, I jumped at the chance!

This was an opportunity for me to leverage my expertise in health and diseases, with nutrition and superfoods, to contribute to both available smoothie recipes, and at the same time to help people suffering with various health issues.

And I hope to expand the scope of this book, covering more diseases and health conditions in the future.

I hope you get some relief while you enjoy these delicious smoothies!

See all the books in the Superfoods Series on my [Amazon's Karen Groves Page](.).

And [drop me a note](.) with your comments – of course your honest review of this book would be most welcome.

INTRODUCTION

People throughout the whole world are dealing with many diseases and health conditions that take joy out of life and even lead to premature death.

For many, changing diet can bring a measure of relief. But completely changing one's diet overnight can be difficult. Making small changes over time is an easier road to travel. ***And introducing smoothies into one's diet can help.***

Smoothies are also an easy way to introduce raw food into one's diet. Why raw food? Raw food has enzymes. There are at least 3,000+ enzymes that we need in our diets, to serve as catalysts for various reactions, to gain and maintain health. There are over 25-30,000 reactions in our bodies that require these enzymes as catalysts to speed up these reactions. Unfortunately, enzymes are destroyed when food is cooked, so we need at least some raw food in our diets for health. Some have even suggested that over 50% of our diets should be raw food. Smoothies and juicing are quick and easy ways to enjoy raw food.

More and more studies and research reveal that diet is one of the major factors in many ailments, and that a truly healthy diet generally will lead to a healthy life, and a poor diet will lead to disease and a lack of health. Even people predisposed to certain health issues will usually fare better with a healthy diet.

This book, part of the Superfoods Series, focuses on 14 diseases and health conditions, and on the superfoods that contain the specific, essential nutrients that play an important role in each of them. Smoothie recipes are then developed that deliver these essential nutrients for each of these 14 health issues.

Specifically, you will find in the following pages 73 smoothie recipes for these diseases and health conditions:

Alzheimer's and Dementia; Arthritis/Rheumatoid Arthritis; Asthma; Cancer; Cholesterol; Depression; Diabetes; Eyesight/Macular Degeneration/Blindness; Fibromyalgia; Gout; Heart Disease/Hypertension (High Blood Pressure); Inflammation; Low Libido/ED and Osteoporosis.

I devote a chapter to each of these health issues, with sections that *describe each health issue* (symptoms, causes, remedies and more); the *role of superfoods*, with lists of fruits, vegetables and other superfoods that carry the nutrients specific to that health issue; and several *smoothie recipes specifically designed to deliver the key nutrients for it*.

In **Conclusion**, I offer some closing thoughts on nutrition and health, and some **Recommended Reads and Resources**.

I also added four appendices on frankly staggering disease statistics, on relationships between the food we eat and our health, on supplementation, and on self-muscle testing:

Appendix I – Disease Statistics

"The following are statistics for the diseases that are included in this book. They help us to realize that these diseases and conditions are found worldwide and the numbers of people dealing with them are increasing. The inclusion of smoothie recipes specifically for each one comes with our hope that they can make a positive difference in the lives of sufferers."

Appendix II – Our Health and Our Food

"The biggest challenge to our health is the food supply. Mass produced food will keep us alive for a time, but will not keep us healthy . . . That is why we see heart disease, diabetes and cancer continuing to rise in spite of medical and governmental recommendations for diet."

Appendix III – Supplementation, considers the need for supplementation to our diets and what supplements to avoid and those to consider

> *"If you question whether or not hard milled supplement tablets actually offer benefit or not, check with your local water purification system and those who handle portable bathrooms . . ."*

Appendix IV – Self-Muscle Testing, shows how to self-muscle test to see if certain foods or supplements can benefit you or should be avoided

> *"Because the tester can sometimes influence the results, if not careful, or there is no one to do the testing, self-muscle testing can be done . . . It's very simple."*

MAKING THE SMOOTHIES

Tips and Suggestions

In this book, I advocate organic superfood where possible and give you smoothie recipes for 14 health conditions. These smoothies are made up mostly of super fruits that supply nutrients that are known to help individuals with a particular health condition or disease. Generally, what I do with these recipes is the following:

1. I start out with a base recipe.

2. I add one or more new ingredients to give you a variation.

My suggestion is that you utilize the recipes up to the point that you feel comfortable and take into consideration your diet. Some of these recipes are rather high calorie, and you may want to drink only 4 ounces and save the rest for later in the day for an afternoon boost. You will be making these smoothies with foods that have fiber, so you should not experience a rush, then a drop in blood sugar, as you would with just straight juice with no pulp. These smoothies should give you needed nutrients and energy as well, without the side effects of sodas.

Feel free to experiment with the ingredient proportions in the smoothies as well. If you like a particular fruit that is included more than another, shift the emphasis. In other words, if you want more pineapple and less banana, make your smoothie that way. Just keep in mind your diet and any health issues involved when you adjust the recipe. (See Life is a Super Fruit for fruit nutritional values.)

Always use chilled juice and fruit. Room temperature just will not cut it. I do not recommend using water ice cubes because they dilute the smoothie, necessitating adding more fruit or sweetener, unless you want one that is more like a slush or snow cone. *Freeze or partially freeze your fruit and any liquid*

that you will be using if you want a slushy type smoothie. You can also add a little more liquid if necessary. Just make sure you have an appliance that can handle frozen fruit and ice cubes.

NOTE: You may not need to freeze the fruit or juice for 24 hours. If you have a freezer that does the job fairly quickly, freeze everything a few hours before making your smoothies.

In some cases, the recipes use a base of fruit juice. ***Use fresh fruit juice (made from the whole fruit) if possible.*** If not, use fruit juice with pulp but no added sugar, and add at least one piece of fresh fruit for the enzymes and fiber. If sugar is a problem, use 50% juice and 50% water.

For those of you that like a less frozen smoothie, you can use frozen fruit and cold milk or juice and make more of a shake rather than a smoothie. During the cold months, I prefer mine like this, but do the more frozen ones during hot weather.

Some of the smoothies may be sweet enough without any additional sweetener; however, I have found that even organic fruit is sometimes more tart than sweet, and a little sweetener helps soften that tartness.

With each disease or condition, I give you a list of fruits and vegetables that help a person deal with that condition. The recipes do not incorporate all of these superfoods. Feel free to experiment with some others on the list. Adding a little bit of ***avocado thickens the smoothie*** and adds a lot of nutrition as well. Because avocado is rather neutral in flavor, it does not take away from the taste of your smoothie.

You can also experiment with making ***green smoothies*** by adding vegetables such as spinach. You can add a little at a time until you get the taste you desire, as well as added nutrition.

You can also ***increase the Vitamin C content*** by adding ¼ teaspoon fresh lemon juice or lime juice to any of the smoothies made with fruit juice, particularly citrus.

A teaspoon of all natural ***peanut butter*** can be added to many of the smoothie recipes as well.

If you find that you are not in love with a particular combination, try adding ½ banana. High in potassium and good taste, bananas seem to pull some ingredients together.

NOTE: A little **cayenne pepper** can be added to smoothies, as cayenne pepper improves circulation. I add it to my smoothies and my scrambled eggs for breakfast. Start with a tiny pinch and gradually add more until you get the taste you desire.

In some cases, I include ***juicing recipes using the veggie superfoods***. Again, you can adjust the proportions of vegetables or even incorporate different ones as well. Just keep in mind that each list of foods is for a particular condition because they have the nutrients that fight those symptoms or nourish the body for maximum defense by strengthening the immune system. Have fun making up your own combinations according to your taste buds and needs. (See [Superfood Vegetables for Health]() for vegetable nutritional values.)

I hope you enjoy the various recipes and experience relief from your symptoms or even find that you no longer have a problem. You may be surprised at what your body can do when properly nourished with superfood smoothies. Enjoy the journey!

Blenders

I frankly recommend a Nutribullet blender.

Nutribullets can handle the frozen cubes and seeds such as flaxseeds, and cost around $100.00. They can handle veggies such as beets as well. I have an older Magic Bullet and was surprised when it made pieces of beets into juice. Since starting this book, I purchased a Nutribullet, and found that it has a much more powerful motor than the original. It makes juice (with added water) of pieces of carrot in a matter of seconds. When you are juicing, however, I would not suggest using as much water as they recommend, because the taste is too diluted. At least it is for my taste. If you do not want to use straight juice as a base, try using 50% juice and 50% water.

NOTE: Nutribullets have the advantage over many conventional juicers in that they keep all of the fiber as well as the nutrients and completely break down the food, even seeds such as flaxseeds. They also have a very powerful motor, and they clean up quickly.

ALZHEIMER'S AND DEMENTIA

About Alzheimer's and Dementia

What are the symptoms of Alzheimer's and Dementia?

Dementia itself is not a disease. Rather, it is a name for a wide range of symptoms. These symptoms include *declines in memory, language and communication skills, ability to pay attention and to focus, judgment and reasoning, visual perception*, or other thinking skills that are severe enough to disrupt and reduce the ability to perform everyday activities. Not every person with dementia will display the symptoms; however having at least two of these severe symptoms would warrant a diagnosis of dementia.

Alzheimer's accounts for about 75% of dementia cases. There are 7 stages of Alzheimer's:

        Stage 1: No impairment

        Stage 2: Very mild decline

        Stage 3: Mild decline

        Stage 4: Moderate decline

        Stage 5: Moderately severe decline

        Stage 6: Severe decline

        Stage 7: Very severe decline

This information, and more detailed information concerning symptoms and stages is available at Alz.org.

What is the cause and cure of Alzheimer's?

The real cause of Alzheimer's is not known; therefore, there is no cure either. There are various medications that seem to alleviate some of the symptoms.

So what can be done to possibly alleviate or prevent the onset of Alzheimer's symptoms?

Since Alzheimer's affects the brain and its functions, nourishing the brain and neurons (nerves) could make a difference.

My mother died in November 2012 at age 94, after 14 years of Alzheimer's. In the beginning she was very anxious, suspicious and convinced someone had entered their house and stolen her property. Unfortunately, she had hidden jewelry, makeup and other of her belongings herself and didn't remember doing so.

Shortly after, she became very aggressive toward those she did not know and even became aggressive toward my father when she no longer recognized him. Before my mother's medication was adjusted to alleviate her aggressive behavior, I would give her 2 ounces of Vemma's Ultra-Premium Antioxidant Supplement. This is a concentrated liquid supplement of vitamins, minerals, mangosteen fruit and aloe. Within an hour my mother would be fine, just as nice as can be. This was her reaction every single time I gave her the supplement. Unfortunately, her doctor said she didn't need a supplement, I had no say in her treatment and those who did agreed with her doctor. As best I can tell my mother died with symptoms of scurvy, a nutritional deficient disease.

I believe that an organic liquid supplement, or superfood smoothies made from whole foods, could help alleviate some of the symptoms of an Alzheimer's patient. In fact, I believe that diet and nutrition may be the key to avoiding or possibly reversing Alzheimer's disease. At this time, because there is no known cause, it is not known if diet can cure Alzheimer's or other forms of Dementia.

Role of Superfoods in Alzheimer's and Dementia

What superfoods might make a difference in prevention of Dementia and Alzheimer's?

Research is finding that certain nutrients do feed and support brain and nerve functions. A number of superfoods have these nutrients and can do this, in addition to supporting the immune system as well. The following are superfoods that may help with Alzheimer's and other dementia because they have nutrients such as potassium, phosphorus, molybdenum, magnesium, choline, iron, omega 3's and saturated fatty acids that feed nerves including those that make up the brain.

Fruits - apples, apricots, avocados, bananas, blueberries, cantaloupe, cherries, figs, grapefruits, grapes, honeydew melons, kiwifruit, lemons, limes, mangos, nectarines, oranges, papaya, peaches, pears, pineapples, plums, pomegranates, raspberries, strawberries and tomatoes – for nutritional values and health benefits of individual super fruits, see Life is a Super Fruit.

Vegetables - beans, broccoli, collard greens, kale, lettuce, mustard greens, onions, sweet potatoes, Swiss chard and turnip greens - for nutritional values and health benefits of individual super veggies, see Superfood Vegetables for Health.

Other - water, chia seeds, coconuts, flaxseeds, dark chocolate, eggs, honey, nuts, red wine, turmeric and organic whole milk yogurt – see The Fats of Life and What You Don't Know Could Kill You and Sometimes You Feel Like a Nut.

NOTE: Drink plenty of good water because you can have the most nutritious diet on the planet, and if you don't drink enough water you will become dehydrated and the nutrients will not get to the cells as they should. And that includes your brain cells. Light to moderate exercise, such as walking, causes the heart to pump more and will help in getting nutrients to the brain as well.

Smoothies for Alzheimer's and Dementia

The following smoothies are targeted to deliver key nutrients for brain and nerve health to help with Alzheimer's and other dementia.

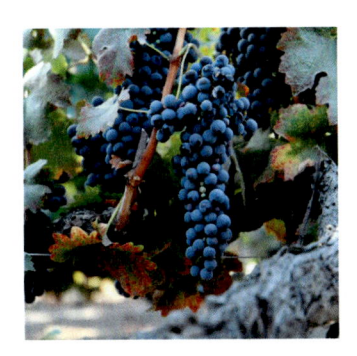

Grapes - Photo by Verita

'I'm In My Right Mind' Smoothie for Brain and Nerve Support

- 4 ounces pomegranate juice

- 4 ounces grape juice

- 1 medium apple

Blend and enjoy - Calories approximately 240

'I'm In My Right Mind' Smoothie – Variation #1

- 4 ounces pomegranate juice

- 4 ounces grape juice

- 1 medium apple

- 1/2 banana

Blend and enjoy - Calories approximately 280

'I'm In My Right Mind' Smoothie – Variation #2

- 8 ounces pomegranate juice
- 1/2 banana
- 1/2 cup mango

Blend and enjoy - Calories approximately 250

'Clear My Mind' Smoothie

- 8 ounces grape juice
- 8 ounces blueberries or mixed berries

Blend and enjoy - Calories approximately 250

'Clear My Mind' Smoothie – Variation #1

- 8 ounces grape juice
- 4 ounces blueberries or mixed berries
- 1/2 banana

Blend and enjoy - Calories approximately 290

'I've Got The Nerve' Smoothie

- 4 ounces orange juice
- 1 medium orange
- 1 medium banana

Blend and enjoy - Calories approximately 200

ARTHRITIS / RHEUMATOID ARTHRITIS

About Arthritis / Rheumatoid Arthritis

What is Arthritis?

Arthritis is *inflammation of one or more joints*. Its symptoms include pain and limited joint function. Arthritis sufferers include men, women and children. Early and accurate diagnosis by a rheumatologist, who is a medical arthritis expert, can help to prevent irreversible joint damage and disability. You can go to MedicineNet.com for articles on Rheumatoid Arthritis, Lupus, Gout, Hip Bursitis, Lyme Disease, and other information concerning arthritis.

There are over 100 different types of arthritis that have been identified, and the medical field is finding more.

In general, arthritis is a joint disorder featuring inflammation and is frequently accompanied by pain. *Osteoarthritis* is a type that causes wear and tear of cartilage, while *rheumatoid arthritis* is associated with inflammation that results from having an overactive immune system. Taken together, *all the different types of arthritis make up the most common chronic illness in the United States*.

Arthritis is classified as one of the rheumatic diseases that separate it from other diseases. All diseases in this classification have a tendency to affect the joints, muscles, ligaments, tendons and cartilage. They may affect other parts of the body as well.

Is fibromyalgia a type of arthritis?

Although it has been called 'arthritis of the muscles', fibromyalgia is not a type of arthritis, as it does not involve the joints. See the chapter on Fibromyalgia for additional information.

What are the causes of arthritis?

There are many different causes of arthritis depending on the type. These include injuries that can lead to osteoarthritis; metabolic abnormalities, such as pseudo-gout and gout; infections, directly or indirectly, due to viruses and bacteria; and misdirected immune systems resulting in rheumatoid arthritis and systemic lupus erythematosus)

Can arthritis be cured?

The medical community will probably say that there is no cure for the various forms of arthritis. For myself, I believe that we are wonderfully made, and if we give our bodies what they need they will do what they should have done in the first place. I see the question in your eyes, "You mean that my body cures itself?" Yes, because there is no doctor, no surgery, no drug, no chemotherapy, no treatment that cures. They can only support the body in healing itself. Any honest health practitioner will tell you the same thing. The trick is to find out 'what' the body needs. And I do feel that diet plays a key role in the healing process.

Role of Superfoods in Arthritis / Rheumatoid Arthritis

If diet is the key, what nutrients can help? Superfoods with vitamin D (essential for joint health), omega-3's (anti-inflammatories) and selenium (nourish cartilage) are among the nutrients that can help alleviate symptoms. Here are the beneficial superfoods:

Fruits - apples, avocados, berries (especially cranberries and blueberries), cherries, grapes, kiwifruit, mangos, pineapples and pomegranates – for nutritional values and health benefits of individual super fruits, see Life is a Super Fruit.

Vegetables - beans; broccoli; Brussels sprouts; cabbage; cauliflower; Crimini mushrooms; dark green, leafy vegetables; kale; onions; red, yellow and orange vegetables – for nutritional values and health benefits of individual super veggies, see Superfood Vegetables for Health.

Other - water, chia seeds, coconuts, eggs, extra virgin olive oil, green tea, nuts, pumpkin and squash seeds, sesame seeds and sunflower seeds – see The Fats of Life and What You Don't Know Could Kill You and Sometimes You Feel Like a Nut.

NOTE: Some who are dealing with arthritis have found it helpful to avoid nightshade plant foods: bell peppers, chili peppers, eggplant, potatoes and tomatoes. This would also include smoking or chewing tobacco.

Here are two web sites you can check out for naturally dealing with arthritis. The first program, Arthritis Interrupted, is by Stephen T. Sinatra, MD and Jim Healthy. This program can help alleviate the symptoms of most types of arthritis. The second program was developed by Clint Paddison, who was suffering from rheumatoid arthritis and who used this program to eliminate his RA symptoms.

Smoothies for Arthritis / Rheumatoid Arthritis

The following smoothies are targeted to deliver key nutrients to help relieve arthritis / rheumatoid arthritis.

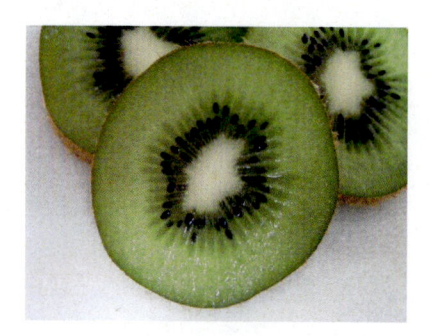

Kiwifruit

'I've Got You Under My Skin' Smoothie for Arthritis

- 8 ounces coconut milk with vanilla

- 1/2 cup mixed berries

Sweeten to taste with honey, sugar or stevia

Blend and enjoy - Calories approximately 170

'I've Got You Under My Skin' Smoothie for Arthritis – Variation #1

- 8 ounces coconut milk with vanilla

- 1/2 cup mixed berries

- 1/2 cup cherries

Sweeten to taste with honey, sugar or stevia

Blend and enjoy - Calories approximately 210

Arthritis Smoothie 2

- 8 ounces coconut milk with vanilla
- 1/2 cup cranberries or ¼ cup cranberry sauce

If using cranberries, sweeten to taste with sugar, honey or stevia

Blend and enjoy - Calories approximately 220 with stevia

Arthritis Smoothie 3

- 8 ounces pineapple juice
- 4 ounces mango

Blend and enjoy - Calories approximately 150

Arthritis Smoothie 3 – Variation #1

- 8 ounces pineapple juice
- 4 ounces mango
- 1/2 cup kiwifruit

Blend and enjoy - Calories approximately 200

Arthritis Smoothie 3 – Variation #2

- 8 ounces pineapple juice
- 4 ounces mango
- 1/2 cup kiwifruit
- 1/2 cup mixed berries

Blend and enjoy - Calories approximately 250

Arthritis Smoothie 4

- 8 ounces pomegranate juice
- 1 medium apple

Blend and enjoy - Calories approximately 200

Arthritis Smoothie 4 – Variation #1

- 8 ounces pomegranate juice
- 1 medium apple
- 1/4 cup cranberry sauce

Blend and enjoy - Calories approximately 250

Arthritis Smoothie 5

- 8 ounces unsweetened cranberry juice
- 1 medium apple

Sweeten to taste with honey, sugar or stevia

Blend and enjoy - Calories approximately 160 if you use stevia

ASTHMA

About Asthma

What is asthma?

Asthma is a chronic lung disorder that is marked by recurring episodes of airway obstruction manifested by labored breathing and accompanied by wheezing, coughing and a sense of constriction in the chest, triggered by hyperactivity or various stimuli such as allergens or rapid changes in air temperature.

There are upwards of 300 million asthmatics worldwide. 250,000 of them will die each year. In the United States alone there are 24.6 million who suffer from asthma, and over 3,000 of these individuals will die each year.

The most common asthma *symptoms include coughing, especially at night, when laughing or from exercise; breathing difficulties; tightness in the chest or feeling of weight on the chest; and wheezing.*

Is asthma a psychological disorder?

No; however, strong emotions from others or even in the asthmatic can adversely contribute to an asthma attack. Especially if the asthmatic panics, the bronchial tubes can constrict causing further reduction of lung capacity. Staying calm can do much towards helping to alleviate an asthma problem or attack.

Is asthma life threatening?

It can be. In fact, since the 1970's the number of asthma cases and deaths has increased significantly. This is why it is important to check with an asthma specialist if you suspect that you or a loved one may have asthma.

What can be done in the case of an asthma attack?

Reflexology: There are acupressure points for the lungs on the bottom of the feet just behind the pads behind the toes, between the toes and the heel. When an asthmatic has trouble breathing, these points can be massaged and can help the bronchial tubes to the lungs to open up so the person can breathe easier. If the asthmatic is not a water drinker, the following might be considered along with massaging the feet.

Encourage the drinking of pure water: Dr. F. Batmanghelidj, MD studied the effects of water and hydration on thousands of patients and found that his asthma patients were dehydrated. Their bodies, in response, were causing an asthma attack in an effort to hang on to the little bit of water left to them. He determined that if he gave them 2 glasses of water and a pinch of sea salt on their tongue that the attack would stop.

He discovered that most of his patients were suffering from dehydration, and when they were hydrated that their symptoms were alleviated no matter what they were dealing with. So, he treated his patients with nothing but water and achieved astonishing results. His web site is WaterCure.com. His book on Asthma and other books can be found on Amazon.com.

Role of Superfoods in Asthma

The following list of superfoods to prevent and alleviate asthma symptoms is from HealWithFood.org. They have specific information as to why these foods can help asthmatics, as well as weekly tips. In general, superfoods help fight inflammation, help prevent constriction of the bronchial tubes and eliminate mucus in the bronchia, as well as strengthen the immune system.

You may find even more benefit from eating organically grown superfoods as they do not have pesticides that may set off asthma symptoms.

Fruits - apples, avocados, bananas, figs (help clear mucus from bronchial tubes), kiwifruit, oranges and tomatoes – for nutritional values and health benefits of individual super fruits, see Life is a Super Fruit.

Vegetables - amaranth leaves, beets, beet greens, broccoli spouts, carrots, endive, kale, mustard greens, okra, onions, spinach, sweet potatoes, turnip greens and winter squash – for nutritional values and health benefits of individual super veggies, see Superfood Vegetables for Health.

Other - water, eggs, flaxseeds, garlic, ginger, rosemary, sesame seeds, sunflower seeds and turmeric – see The Fats of Life and What You Don't Know Could Kill You and Sometimes You Feel Like a Nut.

NOTE: Some have found that pomegranate juice and watermelons have helped their asthma symptoms, but others have found they increased their symptoms. If you choose to try either of these superfoods, use them with care keeping this in mind.

You may want to read these 10 Diet Tips for asthmatics. Also, see

Recipe for Ginger Lemonade

Interesting entry on curezone.com forum

Smoothies for Asthma

The following smoothies are targeted to deliver key nutrients to help relieve the symptoms of asthma.

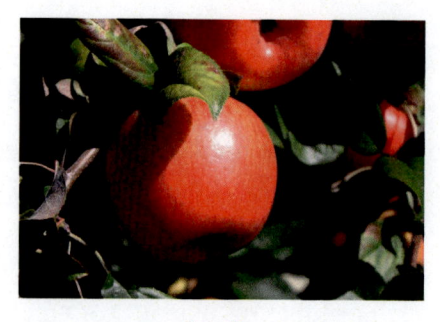

Apples

'Take a Deep Breath' Smoothie for Asthma

- 8 ounces apple juice
- 1 medium apple (for fiber and enzymes)

Blend and enjoy - Calories approximately 180

'Take a Deep Breath' Smoothie for Asthma – Variation #1

- 8 ounces apple juice
- 1 medium apple (for fiber and enzymes)
- 1/2 banana

Blend and enjoy - Calories approximately 230

'Take a Deep Breath' Smoothie for Asthma – Variation #2

- 8 ounces apple juice
- 1 medium apple (for fiber and enzymes)
- 1/2 banana
- 2 reconstituted dried figs

Blend and enjoy - Calories approximately 280

'Take a Deep Breath' Smoothie for Asthma – Variation #3

- 8 ounces apple juice
- 1 medium apple (for fiber and enzymes)
- 1 kiwifruit

Blend and enjoy - Calories approximately 250

Vegetable Smoothie for Asthma #1

- 8 ounces fresh tomato juice
- 1 cup amaranth leaves or beet leaves
- 1 cup spinach

Blend. Add a little more tomato juice if too thick.

Enjoy - Calories approximately 160

Vegetable Smoothie for Asthma #2

- 8 ounces fresh carrot juice
- 1/2 cup kale or spinach leaves
- Pinch of cayenne pepper

Blend and enjoy - Calories approximately 110

CANCER

About Cancer

What is cancer?

Cancer is comprised of over 100 diseases whose characteristics include uncontrolled growth of cells and the ability of these cells to migrate (metastasize) from the original site and spread to other sites. It is easier to beat any cancer before it spreads to other areas of the body.

What are some of the most common cancers?

The most common cancers include: ***Brain cancer, Breast cancer, Bone cancer, Lung cancer, Liver cancer, Stomach cancer, Colon cancer, Prostate cancer, Pancreatic cancer, and Skin cancer.***

What are some of the signs and symptoms of cancer?

The following are some of the indications that a problem may be cancer, but keep in mind that these can also indicate other problems instead: ***unexplained weight loss; persistent fatigue; persistent fever; bowel changes such as constipation, diarrhea or blood in the stool; persistent chronic cough; and pain.***

Can cancer be beaten?

Yes, it can and thousands worldwide are doing just that. However, the medical profession would have us believe that the only way that can be done is through surgery, drug therapy, radiation therapy and chemotherapy. Unfortunately, most people do not realize that chemotherapy destroys the immune system. When that happens, the person may die because they no longer have anything to fight the cancer. My neighbor died after having extensive chemotherapy treatments for lung cancer.

I personally know of an individual who had Hodgkin's disease in the chest area when he was a child. Today, as he ages he deals with scar tissue in his cardiovascular system. He's had to have stent surgery and is on blood thinning medicine. All of this are side effects due to radiation treatments done over 40 years ago.

Conventional treatment may or may not be the answer. Thousands, perhaps millions worldwide, die in spite of conventional treatments. There are hundreds of natural treatments that individuals can utilize that do not have the dangerous side effects of conventional treatments. CancerDefeated.com is just one site that has a lot of information on avoiding cancer and finding natural cancer treatments in addition to survivor experiences.

Why do I say that cancer can be beaten?

First of all, please understand that nobody or no thing such as surgery, drugs or chemotherapy can cure. It is our own bodies that cure. What we have to do is give our bodies what they need to handle the problem, whether it is cancer or something less serious. In the case of cancer, something in one's lifestyle has allowed the few cancer cells, that most of us have in our bodies, to start taking over. This could be a traumatic event, excess stress, diet or environment, among other things. Keeping one's lifestyle in balance as much as possible can go a long way toward preventing cancer growth.

Suzanne Somers and others who have beaten cancer

The actress Suzanne Somers is one individual who was diagnosed with breast cancer and refused conventional treatment with chemotherapy. She looked for and found alternate treatments that have served her well. This site shows an interview with Ms. Somers, Dr. Oz, her breast reconstruction surgeon, and one other doctor concerning her treatment to repair her breast after surgery. I was livid when Ms. Somers said she had agreed with her cancer doctor to have a lumpectomy done and radiation but no chemotherapy, and after the surgery she realized that the doctor had removed 2/3's of her breast when the tumor was very small, about 2cm. Standard procedure is no excuse for that.

If you elect to have any surgery done, make sure you know exactly what the doctor will do and have it **'in writing.'** Do not leave yourself vulnerable to the whim of any medical personnel. It is your body, they are nothing but hired hands, and you have the right to tell them what you want done and what you don't want done. Don't ever fall into the trap of 'that is what we've always done' or 'that is standard procedure.' If your surgeon can't rationalize that 'standard procedure' to your satisfaction, or won't follow your instructions, find another surgeon who will.

Four cancer survivors, each with different types of cancer, are featured at this site summarizing the natural treatments that they used to combat their cancers. If you Google 'cancer survivors and alternative treatment,' you will find over 3 million hits with information. Also, NaturalNews.com/cancer has a number of news stories concerning cancer and cancer treatments you may find of interest.

Role of Superfoods in Cancer

What is one of the major things one can do to help prevent cancer?

Healthy diets, stress management, sleep management and regular exercise, are things that most of us should handle better than we do. Changing over to organic foods as much as possible is one of the biggest positive changes we can make. We really are what we eat, and when we eat a variety of high nutrient foods it can help us deal with the stresses we encounter each day by boosting our immune systems.

In various studies, the following superfoods have shown that they have nutrients that may help prevent or can alleviate the symptoms of various cancers. Some of these nutrients can prevent cancer cells in tumors from multiplying. Others boost the immune system.

Fruits - apples, apricots, bananas, blackberries, cantaloupe, cranberries, grapefruit, grapes, kiwifruit, limes, mangos, nectarines, papayas, peaches, pears, pineapple, plums, raspberries, strawberries, tomatoes and watermelon – for nutritional values and health benefits of individual super fruits, see [Life is a Super Fruit](#).

Vegetables - asparagus, beets, beet greens, Bok choy, broccoli, Brussels sprouts, cabbage, carrots, cauliflower, collard greens, eggplant, kale, mushrooms, okra, onions, peppers (hot), Romaine lettuce, spinach, sweet potatoes, Swiss chard and turnip greens – for nutritional values and health benefits of individual super veggies, see [Superfood Vegetables for Health](#).

Other - water, cayenne pepper, coconuts, coconut milk, flaxseeds, nuts, organic whole milk products (butter, yogurt, sour cream, etc.), sesame seeds and sunflower seeds – see [The Fats of Life and What You Don't Know Could Kill You](#) and [Sometimes You Feel Like a Nut](#).

Smoothies for Cancer

The following smoothies are targeted to deliver key nutrients that may help prevent or can alleviate the symptoms of various cancers.

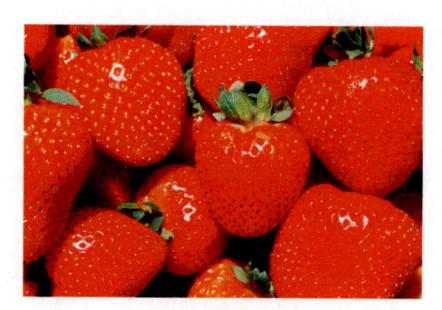

Strawberries

'Never Surrender' Smoothie for conquering Cancer

<u>Never Surrender</u> – **The key message of this song is never give up no matter how tough the situation may be. No matter what happens, no one can ever take away your right to fight. As long as you persevere, nothing's impossible to achieve. The impossible just takes a little longer.**

- 8 ounces unsweetened cranberry juice

- 8 ounces strawberries or mixed berries

Sweeten to taste with sugar, honey or stevia

Blend and enjoy - Calories approximately 160 with stevia

'Never Surrender' Smoothie for conquering Cancer – Variation #1

- 8 ounces unsweetened cranberry juice

- 8 ounces strawberries or mixed berries

- 1 medium apple

Sweeten to taste with sugar, honey or stevia

Blend and enjoy - Calories approximately 250 with stevia

'Never Surrender' Smoothie for conquering Cancer – Variation #2

- 8 ounces unsweetened cranberry juice

- 8 ounces strawberries or mixed berries

- 1 medium banana

Sweeten to taste with sugar, honey or stevia

Blend and enjoy - Calories approximately 240 with stevia

'I Will Survive' Smoothie for kicking Cancer in the butt

Although this song is about going on after a breakup, this attitude can help with the will to live after any situation. Never give up.

- 8 ounces apple juice

- 4 ounces cranberries

Sweeten to taste with sugar, honey or stevia

Blend and enjoy - Calories approximately 110 with stevia

'I Will Survive' Smoothie for kicking Cancer in the butt – Variation #1

- 8 ounces apple juice
- 4 ounces cranberries
- 1 medium banana

Sweeten to taste with sugar, honey or stevia

Blend and enjoy - Calories approximately 200 with stevia

'Eye of the Tiger' Smoothie for kicking Cancer out the door

If you or a loved one is dealing with cancer, it's like looking in the eye of the tiger. And, yes, tigers can be tamed.

- 8 ounces pineapple juice
- 4 ounces coconut milk
- 1/2 cup blackberries

Blend and enjoy - Calories approximately 215

'Eye of the Tiger' Smoothie for kicking Cancer out the door – Variation #1

- 8 ounces pineapple juice
- 4 ounces coconut milk
- 1/2 cup blackberries
- 1/2 medium banana

Blend and enjoy - Calories approximately 260

'Hero' Smoothie for living and loving life

There's always been a hero in your life all along. The hero isn't anyone else – it's you.

- 8 ounces almond milk with vanilla

- 1/2 cup blackberries

Sweeten with honey, sugar or stevia

Blend and enjoy- Calories approximately 135 with stevia

'Hero' Smoothie for living and loving life – Variation #1

- 8 ounces almond milk with vanilla

- 1/2 cup blackberries

- 1/2 banana

Sweeten with honey, sugar or stevia

Blend and enjoy- Calories approximately 180 with stevia

NOTE: For 25 inspirational songs about life and the songs found above, go to **Life**.

CHOLESTEROL

About Cholesterol

What is cholesterol?

Cholesterol is a waxy substance that the body uses for metabolizing sex hormones and fat soluble Vitamins like A, D, E, and K; maintaining cell strength and for repair. About 50% of each cell is made up of cholesterol. (See the section on **More on the Cholesterol Controversy** in the e-book [Superfoods for the Heart](#))

Inflammation in an artery indicates that there is a problem. It could be a rough spot or a potential tear that needs to be repaired. Cholesterol comes along and is utilized like a bandage. Unfortunately, if the inflammation persists, cholesterol continues to be applied until the artery can become partially blocked, causing problems with blood flow. This situation is not because cholesterol is good or bad; it exists because the body has an underlying problem that needs to be addressed. The body's response is inflammation and attempts to repair.

Is having the ideal cholesterol numbers insurance against artery blockage, heart attack or stroke?

No, they aren't because *the size of the cholesterol particles can affect your outcome*. A person can have high cholesterol numbers, and if they have large, fluffy cholesterol particles, they may not have a problem. It is the small, dense cholesterol particles that cause problems because they can get into tiny spaces and continue to accumulate. The larger particles are not able to do that. This probably explains why many people with ideal cholesterol numbers have and die of heart attacks or cancer and many with high cholesterol numbers do not.

But we've been told that high cholesterol, especially the 'bad' cholesterol will kill us.

Well, it isn't the first time we've been conned. ***LDL and HDL are actually designations that let us know which direction cholesterol is moving in relation to the liver***. LDL (low density lipoprotein) actually refers to the carrier combination of cholesterol from the liver to the cells. There is no such thing as LDL cholesterol. HDL (high density lipoprotein) carries cholesterol back to the liver for elimination from the body. If one has small dense cholesterol particles, then having better cholesterol numbers is preferred.

What about statin drugs?

Anyone considering statin drugs because of high cholesterol needs to think twice and get another blood test that will let them know if their cholesterol particles are the small dense ones or the large ones. Then they need to think again because statin drugs carry their own risk. In fact, ALL prescription drugs have side effects, and some of the more popular drugs are actually killing people instead of helping them and putting a lot of money into the pockets of the medical profession and Big Pharma.

Make sure you do plenty of research before saying 'yes' to any drug. There are many effective natural alternatives to taking prescription drugs, and they are cheaper in the long run.

So what can be done to get and keep cholesterol levels in balance?

We keep being bombarded with the terms 'bad' and 'good' cholesterol, however, there is no bad cholesterol. We need cholesterol for health. It just needs to be in the right balance. (See [Superfoods for the Heart and the Cholesterol Controversy](#))

Role of Superfoods in Managing Cholesterol

The following superfoods help balance the HDL and LDL as well as triglycerides (fatty acids circulating in the bloodstream.)

Fruits - avocados, blackberries, blueberries, cranberries, figs, grapefruit, grapes, pears, raspberries and tomatoes – for nutritional values and health benefits of individual super fruits, see Life is a Super Fruit.

Vegetables - amaranth leaves, beets, beet greens, broccoli, Brussels sprouts, cabbage, cucumbers, eggplant, kale, mushrooms (Shitake), okra, onions, peas (green), peppers and romaine lettuce – for nutritional values and health benefits of individual super veggies, see Superfood Vegetables for Health.

Other - water, beef tallow, butter, coconut milk, coconut oil, ghee, lard, nuts, pumpkin and squash seeds, sesame seeds and sunflower seeds – see The Fats of Life and What You Don't Know Could Kill You and Sometimes You Feel Like a Nut.

NOTE: In one study, a group with high cholesterol was given a diet rich in avocados. In one week's time, ALL in the group had balanced cholesterol levels.

Smoothies for Managing Cholesterol

The following smoothies are targeted to deliver key nutrients to help balance your cholesterol.

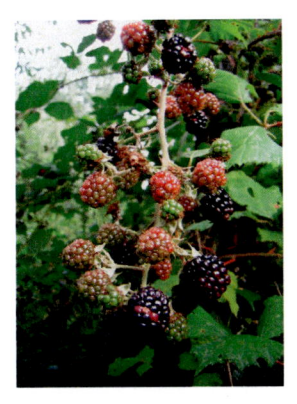

Blackberries

'Music To My Heart' Smoothie for wonderful Cholesterol levels

- 8 ounces coconut or almond milk with vanilla

- 1 cup blackberries or raspberries

Sweeten to taste with honey, sugar or stevia

Blend and enjoy - Calories approximately 170 with stevia

Smoothie for Cholesterol balance #1

- 8 ounces grapefruit juice

- 4 ounces orange or tangerine juice

- 1 small orange or tangerine

- 1/4 teaspoon fresh lemon juice

Sweeten to taste with sugar, honey or stevia if needed

Blend and enjoy - Calories approximately 200 with stevia

Smoothie for Cholesterol balance #2

- 8 ounces grape juice
- 1 cup blackberries
- 1/2 cup pears

Blend and enjoy - Calories approximately 160

DEPRESSION

About Depression

What is depression?

All of us get sad or have the 'blues' for a period of time, but clinical depression is something else entirely. Being sad occasionally doesn't incapacitate us, but Major Depressive Disorder (MDD) does. It can overwhelm and undermine one's ability to lead a normal, active life. Experts compare the effects of MDD to those of diabetes and other chronic diseases.

What are the signs and symptoms of MDD?

Signs are what others see in persons with MDD and symptoms are what the sufferers themselves are experiencing.

Psychological signs and symptoms include the following:

- *Persistent sadness or low mood*
- *Thoughts and feelings of worthlessness*
- *Feelings of self hatred*
- *A feeling of hopelessness*
- *A feeling of helplessness*
- *Feeling like crying*
- *Feelings of guilt*
- *Irritability - even trivial things become annoying*
- *Angry outbursts*
- *Intolerance towards others*
- *Persistent doubting - finding it very hard to decide on things*
- *Finding it impossible to enjoy life*
- *Thoughts of self harm*
- *Thoughts of suicide*

- *Persistent worry*
- *Persistent anxiety*

These signs and symptoms have been taken from MedicalNewsToday.com that also has other information concerning depression and many other diseases and conditions. They also have an article on how using computers at night can cause depression, according to a study on mice and light.

MayoClinic.com also has information on depression symptoms in children and teens.

Role of Superfoods in Depression

Are there foods that can help with the 'blues'?

When we feel down or sad, we may turn to carbohydrates for a lift. Carbohydrates help with depression because they keep serotonin production up. Dark green vegetables and poultry help with serotonin production as well.

The following superfoods may help alleviate symptoms of depression.

Fruits - apricots, avocados, bananas, blackberries, cantaloupe, mangos, oranges, and papaya – for nutritional values and health benefits of individual super fruits, see [Life is a Super Fruit](#).

Vegetables - black beans, broccoli, cabbage chickpeas (garbanzo beans), colorful vegetables, green leafy vegetables, kidney beans, peanuts, pinto beans, white beans and yams – for nutritional values and health benefits of individual super veggies, see [Superfood Vegetables for Health](#).

Other - water, all natural peanut butter, coconut milk, dark chocolate, extra virgin olive oil, flaxseeds, green tea, nuts, parsley, pumpkin seeds, sunflower seeds, turmeric and organic whole milk products (butter, sour cream, cottage cheese, etc.) – see [The Fats of Life and What You Don't Know Could Kill You](#) and [Sometimes You Feel Like a Nut](#).

Smoothies for Depression

The following smoothies are targeted to deliver key nutrients that may help you deal with your blues.

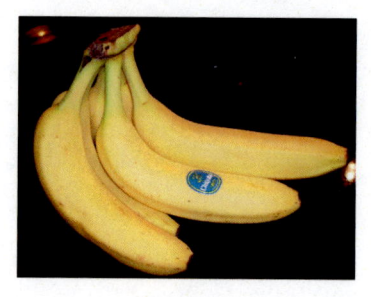

Bananas

'I'm on Top of the World' Smoothie for Depression

- 8 ounces coconut milk

- 1/2 cup mango

Sweeten to taste with honey, sugar or stevia

Blend and enjoy - Calories about 260 with stevia

'I'm on Top of the World' Smoothie for Depression – Variation #1

- 8 ounces coconut milk

- 1/2 cup mango

- 1/2 medium banana

Sweeten to taste with honey, sugar or stevia

Blend and enjoy - Calories about 300 with stevia

'I'm on Top of the World' Smoothie for Depression – Variation #2

- 8 ounces coconut milk
- 1/2 cup mango
- 1/2 medium banana
- 1 tablespoon apricot preserves with no added sugar

Sweeten to taste with honey, sugar or stevia

Blend and enjoy - Calories about 340 with stevia

Smoothie for Depression 2

- 8 ounces orange juice
- 3 apricots or 1 cup canned apricots

Blend and enjoy - Calories approximately 180

Smoothie for Depression 2 – Variation #1

- 8 ounces orange juice
- 3 apricots or 1 cup canned apricots
- 1 medium banana

Blend and enjoy - Calories approximately 260

Smoothie for Depression 2 – Variation #2

- 8 ounces orange juice
- 3 apricots or 1 cup canned apricots
- 1/2 medium banana
- 1/2 cup blackberries

Blend and enjoy - Calories approximately 270

DIABETES

About Diabetes

What is diabetes?

Diabetes is defined as a variable disorder of carbohydrate metabolism caused by a combination of hereditary and environmental factors and usually characterized by inadequate secretion or utilization of insulin; by excessive urine production; by excessive amounts of sugar in the blood and urine; by thirst; hunger and loss of weight.

There are three types of diabetes: Type 1, Type 2 and Gestational (during pregnancy).

Type 1 Diabetes: This type of diabetes can be *congenital or due to injury* and is characterized by a severe lack of insulin. At this time there is no cure. Symptoms of Type 1 are the following: *frequent urination; unusual weight loss; extreme irritability and fatigue; unusual thirst; and extreme hunger.*

Type 2 Diabetes: Type 2 symptoms can be reversed, as *Type 2 is basically a lifestyle disease*. It is important that Type 2 be controlled as it can lead to heart disease, kidney disease, neuropathy and other problems. Symptoms are the following: *Any of Type 1 symptoms; blurred vision; frequent infections; tingling/numbness in feet and hands; cuts or bruises that are slow to heal; and recurring bladder, gum or skin infections.*

Gestational Diabetes: This is experienced by a small number of pregnant women who have high blood glucose levels that may disappear after giving birth; however, it is thought by some researchers that it may be a precursor to developing Type 2 in the future.

Risk factors for gestational diabetes include: *being overweight prior to pregnancy; having had gestational diabetes in a prior pregnancy; and having a family history of diabetes.*

What can be done for Type 2 diabetes other than taking insulin?

Since Type 2 diabetes is a lifestyle issue, changing your diet and your lifestyle can make a major difference. How? Take a look at DeWayne McCulley. He wound up in the hospital with a blood glucose level of 1,337 and in a coma. He reversed his diabetes naturally in 4 months. At the very least, anyone can alleviate at least some of their symptoms.

Role of Superfoods in Diabetes

The following superfoods can help reverse diabetes naturally along with proper diet, stress management, proper sleep and exercise. They contain many nutrients for overall health and fiber that keep blood sugar from spiking after meals.

Fruits - acai berries, apples, artichokes, avocados, blackberries, blueberries, cherries, cranberries, elderberries, figs, grapefruits, grapes, goji berries, kiwifruit, lemons, limes, mangosteen fruit, melons, papaya, peaches, pears, plums, pomegranates, prunes, raspberries, strawberries and tomatoes – for nutritional values and health benefits of individual super fruits, see Life is a Super Fruit.

Vegetables - asparagus, beans (for fiber), beets, Bok choy, broccoli, Brussels sprouts, cabbage, carrots, cauliflower, celery, chickpeas, collard greens, cucumbers, edamame, eggplant (Glycemic Index 15), kale, lentils, mushrooms, okra, onions, peppers, romaine lettuce, spinach, sweet potatoes, turnip greens and zucchini squash – for nutritional values and health benefits of individual super veggies, see Superfood Vegetables for Health.

Other - water, bean sprouts, black tea, chia seeds, chlorella, coconuts, coconut milk, extra virgin olive oil, fish oil, flaxseed oil, flaxseeds, organic dairy, organic eggs, pumpkin and squash seeds, sauerkraut and sea plankton – see The Fats of Life and What You Don't Know Could Kill You and Sometimes You Feel Like a Nut.

Smoothies for Diabetes

The following smoothies are targeted to deliver key nutrients that can help reverse your diabetes.

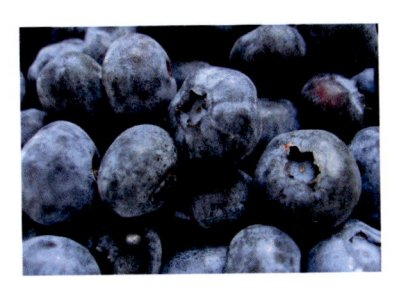

Blueberries

Smoothie #1 for Diabetes

- 8 ounces apple juice

- 1 cup strawberries

Blend and enjoy - Calories approximately 160

Smoothie #2 for Diabetes

- 8 ounces coconut milk with vanilla

- 1 cup blueberries

-1/2 cup strawberries

Sweeten to taste with stevia

Blend and enjoy - Calories approximately 200

Vegetable Smoothie for Diabetes

- 8 ounces carrot juice

- 1 medium tomato

- 1 celery rib

- 1/2 cup fresh spinach

Pinch of cayenne pepper

Blend and enjoy - Calories approximately 200

EYESIGHT/ MACULAR DEGENERATION/ BLINDNESS

About Eyesight/ Macular Degeneration/ Blindness

What is macular degeneration?

Macular degeneration is an eye disorder associated with aging that gradually causes loss of the central vision. There are two types of age-related macular degeneration: dry macular degeneration and wet macular degeneration. Dry macular degeneration is the less severe of the two and usually precedes wet macular degeneration.

What causes macular degeneration?

There is no known cause of this disorder except that it usually comes on with age.

What are the symptoms?

Dry macular degeneration symptoms usually develops gradually. You may notice these vision changes:

- *The need for brighter light when reading or doing close work*
- *Increased difficulty adapting to low light levels, such as when entering a dimly lit restaurant*
- *Increased blurring of printed words*
- *A decrease in the intensity or brightness of colors*
- *Difficulty recognizing faces*
- *A gradual increase in the haziness of your central or overall vision - Crooked central vision*

- *A blurred or blind spot in the center of your field of vision*
- *Hallucinations of geometric shapes or people, in case of advanced macular degeneration*

Dry macular degeneration may affect one or both eyes. If only one eye is affected, you may not notice any changes in your vision because your good eye may compensate for the weak eye.

See your eye doctor if you notice changes in your central vision, or your ability to see colors and fine detail becomes impaired. These changes may be the first indication of macular degeneration, particularly if you're older than age 50.

This information is from MayoClinic.com. Go there for further information about dry and wet macular degeneration and treatments that are available.

What can you do to protect your eyesight?

There are eye exercises and steps you can take to prevent eyestrain when working long hours on the computer. At eye care you will find several videos that will cover some of these steps as well as how to care for your eye wear.

Role of Superfoods in Eyesight/ Macular Degeneration/ Blindness

A well-rounded diet consisting of a number of different foods with plenty of fruits and vegetables can not only help with your eyesight, it can make a great difference to your health overall. Foods high in vitamin A and carotenoids, such as sweet potatoes, carrots, carrot juice, tomato juice, pumpkin, apricots, cantaloupe, spinach, broccoli and leafy green vegetables should be eaten on a regular basis.

Fruit - apples, apricots, blackberries, cantaloupe, cherries, goji berries, grapefruit, kiwifruit, mangos, nectarines, oranges, papaya, peaches, plums, raspberries, strawberries, tomatoes and watermelon – for nutritional values and health benefits of individual super fruits, see Life is a Super Fruit.

Vegetables - beets, broccoli, Brussels sprouts, carrots, collard greens, mustard greens, okra, orange bell peppers, peas (green), pumpkin, romaine lettuce, spinach, squash, sweet potatoes and Swiss chard – for nutritional values and health benefits of individual super veggies, see Superfood Vegetables for Health.

Other - **water,** eggs, fish oils, green tea, nuts, soy and sunflower seeds – see The Fats of Life and What You Don't Know Could Kill You and Sometimes You Feel Like a Nut.

Smoothies for Eyesight/ Macular Degeneration/ Blindness

The following smoothies are targeted to deliver key nutrients that your eyes need, and that can manage, and may even reverse dry macular degeneration.

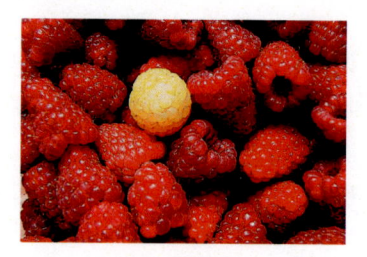

Raspberries

'Better to See You With' Smoothie for good Eyesight

- 8 ounces Almond Milk with Vanilla

- 1/2 medium banana

- 2-4 apricots, 4-6 halves canned apricots in pear juice or 2Tbs apricot preserves with no added sugar

Sweeten to taste with sugar, honey, stevia or 2 ounces of pear juice

Blend, sprinkle nutmeg on top and enjoy - Calories approximately 220 with stevia

'Better to See You With' Smoothie for good Eyesight – Variation #1

- 8 ounces Almond Milk with Vanilla

- 1/2 medium banana

- 2-4 apricots, 4-6 halves canned apricots in pear juice or 2Tbs apricot preserves with no added sugar

- 1/2 cup red raspberries or strawberries

Sweeten to taste with sugar, honey, stevia or 2 ounces of pear juice

Blend and enjoy - Calories approximately 265 with stevia

'Better to See You With' Smoothie for good Eyesight – Variation #2

- 8 ounces Almond Milk with Vanilla

- 1/2 medium banana

- 2-4 apricots, 4-6 halves canned apricots in pear juice or 2Tbs apricot preserves with no added sugar

- 1oz lemonade or 1/2 teaspoon fresh lemon juice for added vitamin C

Sweeten to taste with sugar, honey, stevia or 2 ounces of pear juice

Blend and enjoy - Calories approximately 280 with 1 oz lemonade and stevia

Smoothie for Good Eyesight 2

- 8 ounces orange juice

-3-4 apricots or 2 Tablespoons apricot preserves (no added sugar)

Blend and enjoy - Calories approximately 180

Smoothie for Good Eyesight 3

- 8 ounces apple juice

- 1/2 cup strawberries

- 1/2 cup raspberries

Blend - Calories approximately 180

Veggie Smoothie for Good Eyesight

- 8 ounces fresh carrot juice

- 8 ounces fresh tomato juice

- 1 cup raw spinach

- 1 cup Romaine lettuce

Blend and enjoy - Calories approximately 250

NOTE: You could also add a little ground flaxseed or sunflower seeds. Just make sure that the sunflower seeds are completely pulverized so you don't choke on them when drinking this juice.

FIBROMYALGIA

About Fibromyalgia

What is fibromyalgia?

Fibromyalgia syndrome is soft tissue rheumatism. Rheumatisms are conditions that cause stiffness and pain around joints and in the muscles and bones. Fibromyalgia is different from other rheumatisms in that there is no inflammation, as there is with other rheumatisms, such as bursitis.

Unfortunately, no lab test can confirm a diagnosis of fibromyalgia. Because the syndrome mimics other conditions, diagnosis is determined mainly by trial and error eliminating all others until only fibromyalgia is left.

For a number of years, fibromyalgia was thought to be women's disease and that it was all in their heads. Now it is known that it is a real condition, and it is being diagnosed in men, women and children. Fibromyalgia can be a very debilitating condition in some people preventing them from living a normal lifestyle.

What are the symptoms of fibromyalgia?

There are a number of symptoms that may be experienced by a fibromyalgia sufferer; however, they are intermittent and may show up in different combinations over time. Also, some of the symptoms may indicate other conditions. A healthcare professional has to have a patient keep track of their symptoms over several months so he/she can determine the correct diagnosis. He/she first determines if the patient is experiencing pain on both sides of his body, above and below the waist, for at least 3 months. Other symptoms include the following: ***irritable bowel syndrome, restless leg syndrome, headaches, temporomandibular joint disorder (TMJ), anxiety or***

59

depression, pain in the pelvis, changes in skin color, and sensitivity to temperature and noise.

There are also 18 tender point sites that help to indicate a diagnosis of fibromyalgia. If 11 of these points are tender, it could mean the client has fibromyalgia.

1) *Four spots at the base of the neck, top of the back in a semi-circle*
2) *Inside of the elbows*
3) *Inside of the knees*
4) *Outside top of the thighs*
5) *Either side of the spine at the base of the skull*
6) *Outer lower edges of the collarbone*
7) *Center top of each buttock*
8) *Either side of the windpipe (trachea)*

Because there is no known cause for fibromyalgia, and because of the changeable nature of the symptoms, it can take as long as 5 years to make a correct diagnosis. Those who have already been diagnosed with a rheumatic disease such as rheumatoid arthritis are subject to developing fibromyalgia as well. And as time passes, 90% of patients have fatigue or sleep disturbances that may increase their discomfort.

Role of Superfoods in Fibromyalgia

What can be done to alleviate the symptoms of fibromyalgia?

Regular light exercise and utilizing stress management techniques have proven beneficial to some patients. Many with fibromyalgia are also low in Vitamin D, so getting plenty of sunshine on their skin to produce Vitamin D and eating foods such as mushrooms, organic pork and wild caught fish (like salmon and sardines) can prove helpful. In addition, superfoods that promote serotonin production may make sleep problems less intense.

Fruits – apple, avocados, bananas, cherries (sour), figs, grapes, grapefruit, kiwifruit, melons, peaches, pineapple, plums, prunes, strawberries and watermelon – for nutritional values and health benefits of individual super fruits, see Life is a Super Fruit.

Vegetables - beans, broccoli, Brussels sprouts, cabbage, cauliflower, corn, leafy green vegetables and mushrooms – for nutritional values and health benefits of individual super veggies, see Superfood Vegetables for Health.

Other - water, almonds, brewer's yeast, eggs, flaxseeds, organic whole milk products (butter, cheese, cottage cheese and heavy whipping cream), sesame seeds and sunflower seeds – see The Fats of Life and What You Don't Know Could Kill You and Sometimes You Feel Like a Nut.

Smoothies for Fibromyalgia

The following smoothies are targeted to deliver key nutrients that can be helpful if you suffer from fibromyalgia.

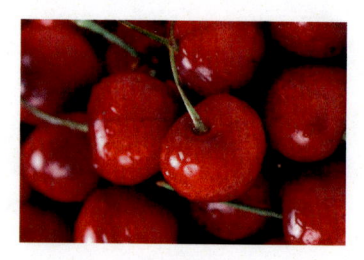

Cherries

Smoothie for Fibromyalgia 1

- 8 ounces pineapple juice
- 1 cup sour cherries

Sweeten to taste with honey, sugar or stevia

Blend and enjoy - Calories approximately 220 with stevia

Smoothie for Fibromyalgia 1 – Variation #1

- 8 ounces pineapple juice
- 1 cup sour cherries
- 1/2 medium banana

Sweeten to taste with honey, sugar or stevia

Blend and enjoy - Calories approximately 260 with stevia

Smoothie for Fibromyalgia 2

- 8 ounces purple grape juice
- 1 cup sour cherries

Sweeten to taste with honey, sugar or stevia

Blend and enjoy - Calories approximately 250 with stevia

Smoothie for Fibromyalgia 2 – Variation #1

- 8 ounces purple grape juice
- 1 cup sour cherries
- 1/2 medium banana

Sweeten to taste with honey, sugar or stevia

Blend and enjoy - Calories approximately 300 with stevia

GOUT

About Gout

What is gout?

Gout is an acute form of arthritis that occurs when uric acid builds up in the blood and causes joint swelling, inflammation and pain. This quite frequently occurs in the big toe but may also affect heel, ankle, elbow, hand or wrist. When uric acid is high, urate crystals settle in the joints and can cause considerable pain. Changes in diet can alleviate the symptoms.

Role of Superfoods in Gout

What can be done for gout flare-ups?

If you are suffering with gout, you need to avoid rich foods and foods high in purines. Purines are broken down into uric acid that can bring on bouts of gout. A list of 224 foods and their purine ratings are found at Acumedico.com.

The following superfoods are low in purines and rich in nutrients.

Fruits - apples, apricots, avocados, bilberries, blueberries, cantaloupe, cherry, currants (red), dried dates, dried figs, gooseberries, grapes, huckleberries, kiwifrut, melons, peaches, pears, pineapple, plums, prunes, raspberries, strawberries and tomatoes – for nutritional values and health benefits of individual super fruits, see Life is a Super Fruit.

Vegetables - asparagus, bean sprouts, beets, broccoli, Brussels sprouts, cabbage, carrots, cauliflower, corn, cucumbers, green beans, kale, mushrooms, peas (green), peppers (green), potatoes with skin, pumpkin, radishes and sauerkraut – for nutritional values and health benefits of individual super veggies, see Superfood Vegetables for Health.

Other - water, aged cheese, all natural peanut butter, Brazil nuts, hazelnuts, organic whole milk and whole milk products (cottage cheese, sour cream, etc), peanuts, tofu and walnuts – see [The Fats of Life and What You Don't Know Could Kill You](#) and [Sometimes You Feel Like a Nut](#).

Smoothies for Gout

The following smoothies are targeted to deliver key nutrients that can help you avoid gout flare-ups.

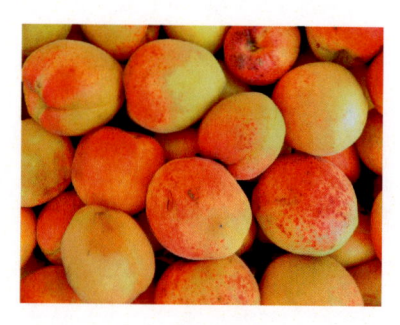

Apricots

'Toe the Line' Smoothies for Gout

- 8 ounces purple grape juice

- 1 medium apple

Blend and enjoy - Calories approximately 170

'Toe the Line' Smoothies for Gout – Variation #1

- 8 ounces purple grape juice

- 1 medium apple

- 1 cup apricots or bilberries, or 2 tablespoons apricot or bilberry preserves

Blend and enjoy - Calories approximately 260

'Toe the Line' Smoothies for Gout – Variation #2

- 8 ounces purple grape juice
- 1 medium apple
- 1 cup mixed berries

Blend and enjoy - Calories approximately 260

Smoothie for Gout 2

- 8 ounces pineapple juice
- 1 cup mixed berries
- 1 Tablespoon apricot or bilberry preserves

Blend and enjoy - Calories approximately 260

HEART DISEASE/ HYPERTENSION/ STROKE

About Heart Disease/ Hypertension/ Stroke

What is heart disease?

The following is the definition of heart disease, symptoms and signs of heart attack according to the staff at the Mayo Clinic.

"Heart disease is a broad term used to describe a range of diseases that affect your heart. The various diseases that fall under the umbrella of heart disease include diseases of your blood vessels, such as coronary artery disease; heart rhythm problems (arrhythmias); heart infections; and heart defects you're born with (congenital heart defects).

The term "heart disease" is often used interchangeably with "cardiovascular disease." Cardiovascular disease generally refers to conditions that involve narrowed or blocked blood vessels that can lead to a heart attack, chest pain (angina) or stroke. Other heart conditions, such as infections and conditions that affect your heart's muscle, valves or beating rhythm, are also considered forms of heart disease.

Many forms of heart disease can be prevented or treated with healthy lifestyle choices."

What are some of the symptoms of heart disease?

The following symptoms are taken from WebMD.com, where you can also find more detailed information concerning the various diseases affecting the heart.

The most common *symptom of coronary artery disease* is angina, or chest pain. Angina can be described as a discomfort, heaviness, pressure, aching, burning, fullness, squeezing, or painful feeling in your chest. It can be mistaken for indigestion or heartburn. Angina may also be felt in the shoulders, arms, neck, throat, jaw, or back. Other symptoms of coronary artery disease include:

- *Shortness of breath*
- *Palpitations (irregular heart beats)*
- *A faster heartbeat*
- *Weakness or dizziness*
- *Nausea*
- *Sweating*

Symptoms of a heart attack can include:

- *Discomfort, pressure, heaviness, or pain in the chest, arm, or below the breastbone*
- *Discomfort radiating to the back, jaw, throat, or arm*
- *Fullness, indigestion, or choking feeling (may feel like heartburn)*
- *Sweating, nausea, vomiting, or dizziness*
- *Extreme weakness, anxiety, or shortness of breath*
- *Rapid or irregular heartbeats*

What can be done to protect your heart?

You can live a lifestyle that includes regular exercise, adequate sleep, healthy eating, and stress management. You can also avoid things such as smoking; recreational drugs; prescription drugs where possible; alcohol abuse; anger and violent music, games or movies. Get together with family and friends. Do things you love and help others as well.

Laugh a lot. Laughter is a great medicine. Norman Cousins was diagnosed with a potentially fatal disease, but he beat the odds. He found that large doses of laughter really did turn out to be great medicine. His book Anatomy of an Illness can be found at Amazon.com.

And pay attention to what you eat, as suggested in the next section.

Role of Superfoods in Heart Disease

Here are the superfood do's and don'ts for your heart health.

Avoid refined, polyunsaturated oils like canola, cottonseed, safflower, soybean and sunflower. Avoid hydrogenated foods of any kind. Avoid fast food and highly processed foods. Eat natural, organic and wild caught foods.

For more information concerning food and your heart, go to:

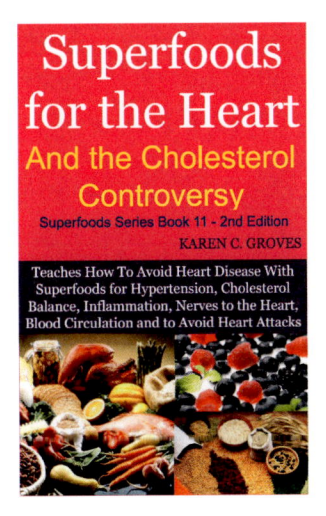

The following superfoods can help with heart health by feeding the nerves to the heart, promoting good circulation, helping with normal heartbeat and boosting your overall health in general.

Fruits - acai berries, apples, apricots, avocados, bananas, blackberries, blueberries, cantaloupes, cherries, figs, goji berries, grapefruits, grapes, guava, honeydew melons, kiwifruit, lemons, limes, mangos, mangosteen fruit, nectarines, oranges, papaya, peaches, pears, pineapple, plums, raspberries, strawberries, tangerines, tomatoes and watermelon – for nutritional values and health benefits of individual super fruits, see Life is a Super Fruit.

Vegetables - amaranth leaves, asparagus, beans, beets, beet greens, Bok choy, broccoli, Brussels sprouts, cabbage, carrots, cauliflower, celery, collard greens, cucumbers, eggplant, green beans, kale, mushrooms (Shitake), mustard greens, okra, onions, peas (green), peppers, pumpkins, romaine lettuce, spinach, squash, sweet potatoes, Swiss chard, turnip greens and yellow corn (organic, not GMO) – for nutritional values and health benefits of individual super veggies, see Superfood Vegetables for Health.

Other - water, animal fat (surprise?), cayenne pepper, chia seeds, cinnamon, coconut milk, coconut oil, dark chocolate, eggs, extra virgin olive oil, flaxseeds, garlic, ginger, ginkgo biloba, green tea, hibiscus tea, maca, nuts, olives, organic whole milk, organic whole milk products, paprika, parsley, pumpkin and squash seeds, red palm oil, red wine, sunflower seeds, turmeric, unrefined walnut oil, wheat grass and yeast – see The Fats of Life and What You Don't Know Could Kill You and Sometimes You Feel Like a Nut.

Smoothies for Heart Health

The following smoothies are targeted to deliver key nutrients that can improve your heart health.

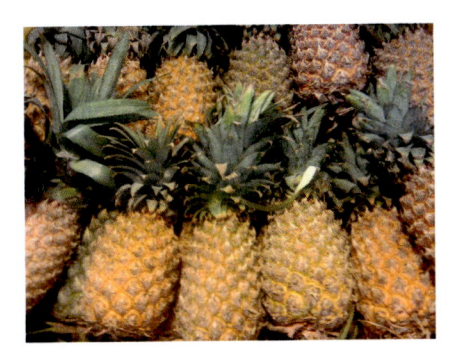

Pineapple

'Virgin Piña Colada' Smoothie for Heart Health

- 2/3 cup pineapple juice

- 1/3 cup coconut milk

- 2-3 drops of vanilla extract

Sweeten to taste with honey, sugar or stevia.

Blend frozen pineapple juice and coconut milk until smooth. If it is too thick, thin with a little pineapple juice. Makes about 1 1/2 cups at about 200 calories, give or take a little, depending on whether or not you add additional sweetener. Enjoy.

NOTE: There is also a French Vanilla Coconut Milk Creamer (Dairy Free) that is great with pineapple juice. It is 20 calories per tablespoon, and that should be considered when making your smoothie, as the creamer is sweetened with dried cane syrup. You definitely will NOT need to add sweetener.

'Virgin Piña Colada' Smoothie for Heart Health - Variation

- 2/3 cup pineapple juice

- 1/3 cup coconut milk

- 2-3 drops of vanilla extract

- 1/2 banana or 1/2 cup strawberries

Sweeten to taste with honey, sugar or stevia.

Blend frozen pineapple juice and coconut milk until smooth. If it is too thick, thin with a little pineapple juice. Makes about 1 1/2 cups at about 250 calories, give or take a little, depending on whether or not you add additional sweetener. Enjoy.

'My Blue Heaven' Coconut Smoothie for Heart Health

- 8 ounces coconut milk

- 1/2 cup blueberries

Sweeten to taste with honey, sugar or stevia

Blend coconut milk and blueberries. Add just a little more coconut milk if needed to blend. Blend and enjoy - Calories about 250 with stevia

'My Blue Heaven' Coconut Smoothie for Heart Health – Variation #1

- 8 ounces coconut milk
- 1/2 cup blueberries
- 1/2 medium banana

Sweeten to taste with honey, sugar or stevia

Blend coconut milk and blueberries. Add just a little more coconut milk if needed to blend. Blend and enjoy - Calories about 330 with stevia

'My Blue Heaven' Coconut Smoothie for Heart Health – Variation 2

- 8 ounces coconut milk
- 1/2 cup blueberries
- 1/2 medium banana
- 1 tablespoon apricot preserves with no added sugar

Sweeten to taste with honey, sugar or stevia

Blend coconut milk and blueberries. Add just a little more coconut milk if needed to blend. Blend and enjoy - Calories about 370 with stevia

'My Blue Heaven' Coconut Smoothie for Heart Health – Variation 3

- 8 ounces coconut milk
- 1/2 cup blueberries
- 1/2 medium banana
- 1 tablespoon apricot preserves with no added sugar
- 1/2 medium mango with skin

Sweeten to taste with honey, sugar or stevia

Blend coconut milk and blueberries. Add just a little more coconut milk if needed to blend. Blend and enjoy - Calories about 430 with stevia (This smoothie you might want to split into 2 servings several hours apart.)

INFLAMMATION

About Inflammation

What is inflammation?

Inflammation is a diseased condition produced in a tissue, organ or body part by an infection, injury or irritant that is characterized by heat, redness, swelling and pain. It is the body's response to indicate there is a problem that needs to be corrected. When the problem is corrected (healed), the inflammation disappears.

There are 3 stages of inflammation:

1) *<u>Vasodilation</u> - the blood vessels dilate allowing increased blood flow to the injured area to increase nutrients and oxygen for healing*
2) *<u>Migration</u> of white blood cells (phagocytes) to the site to ingest any dying or dead tissue, foreign material or bacteria*
3) *<u>Repair</u> with growth of new tissue and restoring normal function to the area*

It is thought by some that inflammation is the root cause of disease, particularly of heart disease, and the problems with cholesterol.

What can be done in regard to inflammation?

There are several steps that you can take to avoid inflammatory responses:

- *Avoid any injury as much as possible*
- *Avoid refined foods, especially oils*
- *Avoid hydrogenated foods*
- *Avoid trans fats*

- *Avoid foods high in omega 6's - Eat foods with a more 1:1 ratio (no more than 1:3 ratio) of omega 3's to omega 6's*
- *Avoid GMO (Genetically Modified Organisms), GE (Genetically Engineered) or any modified food of any kind, including Frankenfish*
- *Live a lifestyle that will allow you to be as healthy as possible.*
- *Make sure you have a wide enough range of food for all nutrients, especially Vitamin C. Take liquid whole organic food supplements (organic minerals with fulvic acid) to fill any gaps in nutrition.*

Role of Superfoods in Inflammation

The following superfoods could make a difference in keeping inflammation under control. Also, making sure you have enough vitamin C in your diet is important, as our bodies make all vitamins EXCEPT vitamin C. Having enough vitamin C will help prevent symptoms of scurvy from developing. (See the section: ***More on the Cholesterol Controversy*** and the comments of Dr. Matthias Rath concerning scurvy-heart disease, in the book Superfoods for the Heart). Always eat natural, organic or wild caught foods where possible.

Fruits - acai berries, apples, avocados, blackberries, blueberries, cherries, citrus fruits, goji berries, grapes, kiwifruit, mangos, oranges, papaya, pineapple, pomegranate juice, raspberries, strawberries and tomatoes – for nutritional values and health benefits of individual super fruits, see Life is a Super Fruit.

Vegetables - amaranth leaves, asparagus, beans, broccoli, Brussels sprouts, cabbage, carrots, cauliflower, collard greens, cucumbers, edamame, green beans, hot peppers, kale, lettuce, mustard greens, okra, onions, radishes, romaine lettuce, spinach, Swiss chard, turnip greens and winter squash – for nutritional values and health benefits of individual super veggies, see Superfood Vegetables for Health.

Other - water, all natural peanut butter, almonds, basil, cayenne pepper, chia seeds, cloves, coconut oil, dark chocolate, extra virgin olive oil, flaxseeds, garlic, ginger, green tea, hot peppers, red wine, organic soy beans, tofu, turmeric and walnuts – see The Fats of Life and What You Don't Know Could Kill You and Sometimes You Feel Like a Nut.

Smoothies for Inflammation

The following smoothies are targeted to deliver key nutrients that can help keep your inflammation under control.

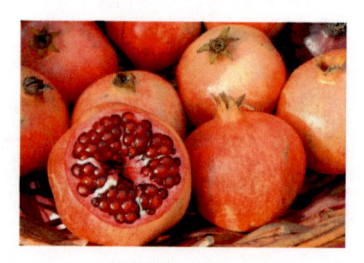

Pomegranates
Photo by Flickr Government Press Office

Smoothie for Inflammation 1

- 8 ounces cherry juice

- 1/2 cup blackberries

Sweeten to taste with honey, sugar or stevia

Blend and enjoy - Calories approximately 245 with stevia

Smoothie for Inflammation 2

- 8 ounces pomegranate juice

- 1 cup strawberries

Blend and enjoy - Calories approximately 240

Vegetable Smoothie for Inflammation

- 8 ounces fresh tomato juice

- 1/2 cup romaine lettuce or spinach

Blend and enjoy - Calories approximately 140

LOW LIBIDO/ ERECTILE DYSFUNCTION

About Low Libido/ Erectile Dysfunction

What is libido?

One dictionary defines libido as sexual desire or impulse: the instinctual craving or drive behind all human activities.

"Having a sex drive and being able to enjoy it isn't all there is to life, but it enhances life, especially between two people who love each other. Sex isn't just about procreation; it is about getting close to another human being in a physical way. This is very important because after the children are grown and leave the nest, a couple should be able to enjoy one another's companionship. They need to grow closer together mentally and emotionally, especially if they intend to spend the rest of their lives together. Having a great sex life can help with that bonding." (Quote from Eat Your Way to Great Sex)

Health and sex go hand in hand. A healthy person has a good libido; an unhealthy person may not be able to perform sexually or may not even have an interest in sex. Because people are living longer (into their 90's or 100's), a couple needs to be as healthy as possible in order to enjoy that life and each other.

What is low libido?

Low or no sexual desire is considered low libido.

USA Today brought out that "20-30% of men and 30-50% of women say they have little or no sex drive."

Did you know that ***Newsweek*** reported that 15-20% of couples had sex about 10 times a year and that this is considered a sexless marriage?

10% of men worldwide experience erectile dysfunction (ED) and the numbers are increasing.

What can cause low libido or poor performance in men?

Aging seems to cause poorer performance for some; however, even younger individuals are beginning to experience low libido and poor performance. So the cause has to be something else. In all probability it is lifestyle: stress, lack of sleep, illness, medications and especially diet.

Erectile dysfunction (impotency) is usually caused by one or more of the following:

- *Age*
- *Type 2 diabetes or other underlying disease*
- *High blood pressure*
- *Loss of sleep*
- *Depression*
- *Anxiety and stress*
- *Problems in relationship*
- *Sexually transmitted diseases*
- *Eating foods that lower libido and fertility*
- *Environmental contaminants*
- *Poor diet overall*
- *Obesity*
- *Abuse of alcohol*
- *Smoking*
- *Substance abuse*

Role of Superfoods in Libido/ Erectile Function

The following superfoods can help with libido and sexual performance. And for more information about superfoods for Improved Libido: Desire, Fertility, Energy, Erectile Function and Great Orgasms, see:

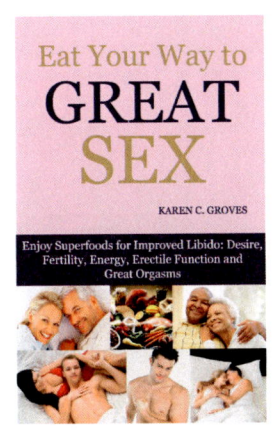

Fruits - acai berries, avocados, bilberries, blackberries, blueberries, dates, figs, goji berries, oranges, pineapple, pomegranates, raspberries and strawberries – for nutritional values and health benefits of individual super fruits, see Life is a Super Fruit.

Vegetables - asparagus, bell peppers, black beans, carrots, celery, chickpeas, chili peppers, leafy greens, peanuts, romaine lettuce and sweet potatoes – for nutritional values and health benefits of individual super veggies, see Superfood Vegetables for Health.

Other - water, all natural peanut butter, almonds, Brazil nuts, coconut oil, eggs, foods high in Vitamin A, garlic and organic whole milk products – see The Fats of Life and What You Don't Know Could Kill You and Sometimes You Feel Like a Nut.

Smoothies for Libido and Erectile Function and More

The following smoothies are targeted to deliver key nutrients that can help your libido and sexual performance.

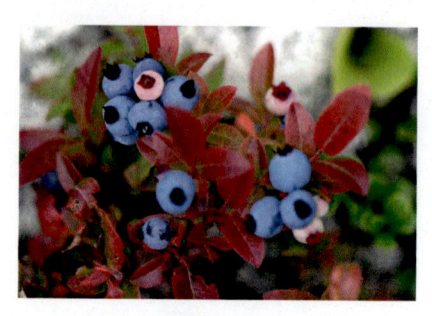

Bilberries

Smoothie for Low Libido/ ED/ Low Fertility

- 8 ounces pineapple juice

- 1 cup bilberries or blueberries

Blend and enjoy - Calories approximately 220

Smoothie for Low Libido/ ED/ Low Fertility - Variation

- 8 ounces pineapple juice

- 1 cup bilberries or blueberries

- 1 teaspoon coconut oil

Blend and enjoy - Calories approximately 260

Smoothie for Low Libido/ ED 2

- 8 ounces pomegranate juice
- 1 cup blueberries

Blend and enjoy - Calories approximately 240

Smoothie for Low Libido/ ED 2 - Variation

- 8 ounces pomegranate juice
- 1 cup blueberries
- 2 dried figs

Blend and enjoy - Calories approximately 290

Smoothie for Low Libido/ ED 3

- 8 ounces orange juice
- 1 cup blueberries

Blend and enjoy - Calories approximately 180

Smoothie for Low Libido/ ED 3 - Variation

- 8 ounces orange juice
- 1 cup blueberries
- 1/2 teaspoon coconut oil

Blend and enjoy - Calories approximately 200

OSTEOPOROSIS

About Osteoporosis

What is osteoporosis?

The word osteoporosis means 'porous bones' and refers to bones that lose density over time and therefore promote fractures. Approximately 50% of women age 50 and over will experience fractures related to osteoporosis.

Most will not even know that they have osteoporosis until they experience a fracture or have a change in posture indicating loss of bone in their spines. During one's lifetime, bone is constantly being rebuilt. Eventually, there is more bone lost than is replaced.

NOTE: A number of facts and statistics can be found at International Osteoporosis Foundation.

Why do we see osteoporosis on the rise?

Very likely, adhering to low-fat diets is part of the problem. Why do I say that?

Calcium and vitamin D are the two main nutrients needed for strong bones. Calcium absorption is dependent on the presence of vitamin D; however, Vitamin D is a fat soluble vitamin that requires saturated fat for it to be utilized. Low fat milk and milk products may have calcium and vitamin D but not enough saturated fat for them to be utilized for bone repair/growth.

Research is indicating that many people are deficient in vitamin D. This deficiency could be due to a lack of sufficient saturated fat in the diet, the use of sunscreens that do not allow the body to utilize the sun's rays so the skin will produce vitamin D, and too low a level of cholesterol in the skin for vitamin D production. Take your pick! All of the above? Probably, each of these contributes to osteoporosis.

What can be done to prevent or alleviate the symptoms of osteoporosis?

Eating a healthy diet, doing weight bearing exercise and getting vitamin D from sunshine as well as food is a must even for young people if they are to avoid osteoporosis after age 50.

Role of Superfoods in Osteoporosis

What can be done to prevent or alleviate the symptoms of osteoporosis?

The following superfoods can help, and can go a long way toward being part of a healthy lifestyle.

Fruits - avocados, blackberries, blueberries, cranberries, pears, raspberries, red grapefruit, strawberries, tomatoes and watermelon – for nutritional values and health benefits of individual super fruits, see Life is a Super Fruit.

Vegetables - asparagus, beans, Bok choy, broccoli, collard greens, kale, mustard greens, peanuts, spinach and turnip greens – for nutritional values and health benefits of individual super veggies, see Superfood Vegetables for Health.

Other, water, all natural peanut butter, almonds, animal fat, Brazil nuts, coconut oil, flaxseeds, hard cheese, organic fortified whole milk, organic whole milk yogurt, tofu and walnuts – see The Fats of Life and What You Don't Know Could Kill You and Sometimes You Feel Like a Nut.

Smoothies for Osteoporosis

The following smoothies are targeted to deliver key nutrients that can help prevent or alleviate the symptoms of osteoporosis.

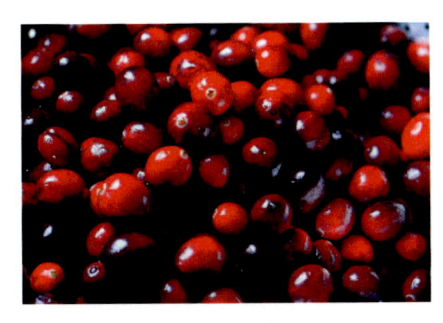

Cranberries

Smoothie for Osteoporosis 1

- 8 ounces cranberry juice

- 1 cup blueberries

Sweeten to taste with honey, sugar or stevia

Blend and enjoy - Calories approximately 160 with stevia

Smoothie for Osteoporosis 2

- 8 ounces cranberry juice

- 1 cup blackberries

Sweeten to taste with honey, sugar or stevia

Blend and enjoy - Calories approximately 160 with stevia

CONCLUSION

Raw superfood smoothies are a great way to add a lot of nutrition to one's lifestyle. At the end of the day, when all is said and done, it appears that diet is the main disease culprit. Eating organic, natural, grass-fed and wild caught food could mean the difference between living a long life relatively free of health issues, or living a life fraught with disease or even having one's life shortened prematurely due to disease and not accident.

In the United States, we have been told healthy eating means eating 'low fat'; however, the 50+ years that Americans have been eating low fat has seen an increase in degenerative diseases rather than a decline. It should be obvious after this long a period of time that 'low fat' doesn't work. In the 50's, President Eisenhower had a heart attack and was put on a low fat diet. He eventually died of heart disease. The low fat diet didn't change a thing as far as alleviating his heart disease.

Low cholesterol levels have been touted as being healthy, yet research is showing that even though many individuals with low cholesterol don't die of heart disease, they die of cancer instead. They just replace one killer with another.

Saturated animal fat has been blamed for heart disease but that is not true. Check out this quote from Dr. Mary Enig's article [The Truth about Saturated Fats](#).

> "A chorus of establishment voices, including the American Cancer Society, the National Cancer Institute and the Senate Committee on Nutrition and Human Needs, claims that animal fat is linked not only with heart disease but also with cancers of various types. Yet when researchers from the University of Maryland analyzed the data they used to make such claims, they found that **vegetable fat consumption** was correlated with cancer and animal fat was not." (Our emphasis)

And then there was the other Alzheimer's patient in the room with my mother. Every day she would demand pudding and Coca Cola, and the caretakers would give it to her. Yes, she was dealing with Alzheimer's, but she had something going for her because she was 108 years of age, giving an indication that diet might not be all there is to the story.

Norman Cousins wrote a book about winning the war against his disease in ***Anatomy of an Illness*** by using laughter and supplements. He took charge of his own health and won. He also realized that the mind is a powerful thing. You will find it interesting to read of the interview with Norman Cousins about [positive emotions and health](). Especially of interest is the placebo study where they did NOT use a placebo. The results were very interesting.

In the final analysis, all of us should take charge of our health, do research and determine how we personally can get and stay healthy. Superfood smoothies can help, but they are not the total solution. Lifestyle consisting of healthy diet, exercise, adequate sleep, stress management, laughter and realizing how powerful we are mentally and emotionally can go a long way in helping us attain a measure of health and, barring accident, a long life.

May you and your loved ones succeed in finding the health and happiness that everyone on this wonderful planet should have available to them.

RECOMMENDED READS AND RESOURCES

Here are some other interesting Kindle e-books for you, with great smoothie recipes:

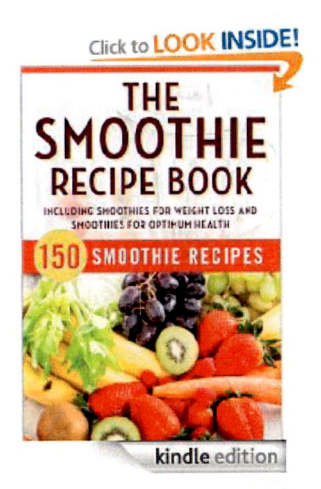

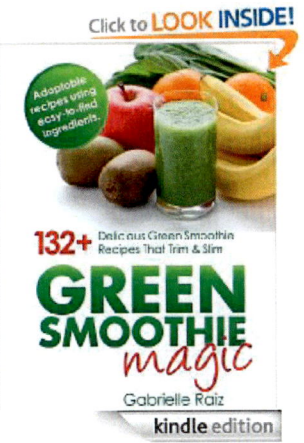

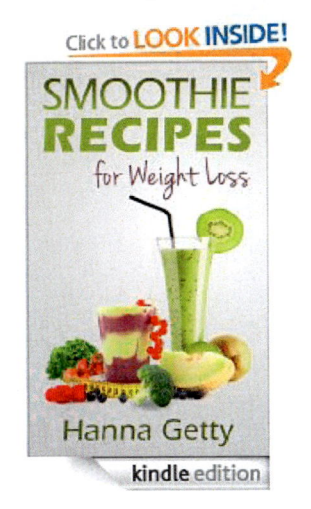

And here is my entire Superfoods Series, to date, with more on the way:

The Superfoods Series

Book 1 – Life is a Super Fruit

Book 2 – Superfood Vegetables for Health

Book 3 – Superfoods Meat, Fish and Seafood for Health

Book 4 – Superfood Legumes for Health

Book 5 – Superfood Grains for Health

Book 6 – Sometimes You Feel Like a Nut

Book 7 – The Fats of Life and What You Don't Know Could Kill You

Book 8 – Superfood Specialty Foods for Health

Superfoods Series Supplement – Superfood Fruit Health Benefits

Eat Your Way to Great Sex

Superfoods for the Heart and the Cholesterol Controversy

Vegetarian Superfoods Package

Smoothies Targeted for Specific Health Issues

Superfoods for the Brain

Here are links to some more in-depth information:

Article by one of the world's top authorities on fats - [The Truth about Saturated Fats](#) - includes information about other fats as well.

For a 100-year chronological history of heart disease, go to [heart disease](#).

Article and study info about starting the day with [fats](#)

Video on what types of food to eat to [lose weight](#)

[Amazing Coconut Oil](#) by Karen McKay at Amazon.com

[The Palm Oil Miracle](#) by Dr. Bruce Fife at Amazon.com - Studies cited show the benefits of red palm oil and the poor results of other oils such as canola and soybean.

Article [The Best You Can Buy](#) in regard to coconut oil

Article on [Dangers of GMO Foods](#)

[OmegaNutrition.com](#) has cold pressed oils in opaque packaging.

To get more information concerning fulvic acid and its benefits, go to [Fulvic](#).

[Prescription for Nutritional Healing](#) at Amazon.com

APPENDIX I – DISEASE STATISTICS

The following are statistics for the diseases that are included in this book. They help us to realize that these diseases and conditions are found worldwide and the numbers of people dealing with them are increasing. The inclusion of smoothie recipes specifically for each one comes with our hope that they can make a positive difference in the lives of sufferers.

Alzheimer's/Dementia - "As of 2010, there are an estimated 35.6 million people with dementia worldwide. This number will double about every 20 years to an estimated 65.7 million in 2030, and 115.4 million in 2050." - From article on Alzheimer's Disease International's web site

Arthritis/Rheumatoid Arthritis - Information taken from Terraclouds.com shows at least 548 million suffer worldwide from some type of arthritis. Statistics, in reality, are probably much higher because these statistics only reflect 15 countries in 2004.

Asthma Facts

- *Estimates are that from 235-300 million people suffer from asthma worldwide.*
- *Asthma is the most common chronic disease among children.*

Cancer - In 2008, an estimated 12.6 million people were diagnosed with some form of cancer and over 7 million died. These cancers included female breast cancer, lung and stomach cancer. (Statistics are from the ***The World Cancer Factsheet*** found at CancerResearchUK.org)

Cholesterol - There continues to be conflicting information concerning whether or not high cholesterol numbers are causing heart disease. See the section ***More on the Cholesterol Controversy*** in The Fats of Life and What You Don't Know Could Kill You.

Depression - "Depression affects 121 million people worldwide. It can affect a person's ability to work, form relationships, and can destroy their quality of life. At its most severe, depression can lead to suicide and is responsible for 850,000 deaths every year." - Biomedcentral.com

Diabetes - "Diabetes is a leading threat to global health and development. According to IDF, the disease now affects over 300 million people worldwide and will cost the global economy at least US$376 billion in 2010, or 11.6% of total world healthcare expenditure. A further 344 million people are at risk of developing type 2 diabetes, the most common form of the disease. If nothing is done to reverse the epidemic, IDF predicts that by 2030, 438 million people will live with diabetes at a cost projected to exceed US$490 billion." - International Diabetes Federation .

Eyesight/Macular Degeneration/Blindness - "Approximately 800 million people worldwide are blind, severely visually impaired or have near vision sight loss according to estimates by the International Agency for the Prevention of Blindness (information from CIBA Vision)

Fibromyalgia – Estimates are that 200-400 million people worldwide suffer from fibromyalgia syndrome. It is not just women's disease, as it strikes men and children as well.

Gout - Approximately 2 in 363 persons, or 0.28%, or 748,000 in the United States are subject to gout. Extrapolated statistics for most countries are found at RightDiagnosis.com. (Extrapolated can mean educated guesstimates or SWAG's - Scientific Wild Ass Guesses. And they do warn you.)

Heart Disease - An estimated 17 million deaths worldwide are due to cardiovascular disease. Many of these deaths were due to heart attacks and strokes. - Statistics are from WHO (World Health Organization)

Inflammation - Inflammation itself is an immune response by the body in an effort to heal. It can be in response to an injury or a disease. Many researchers are beginning to suspect that inflammation is a precursor to degenerative diseases. There are no worldwide statistics except for specific diseases such as inflammatory breast cancer or PID (pelvic inflammatory disease.)

Low Libido/ED - It has been estimated that at least 10% of men worldwide have ED (erectile dysfunction) and the numbers are rising. 30-50% of women admit they have little or no sex drive.

Osteoporosis - Osteoporosis affects an estimated 75 million people in Europe, USA and Japan. However, it is estimated that 200 million women worldwide are affected by osteoporosis.

APPENDIX II – OUR HEALTH AND OUR FOOD

Understanding possible causes of disease and what certain foods can do to alleviate the symptoms can go a long way to give relief and, in some cases, allow the body to heal itself. To heal itself? Yes, because there is no medicine, no surgery, no medical personnel, chemotherapy, radiation or other procedure that actually heals. When we give our body what it needs, it can function the way it should to keep us healthy, and can heal itself. When our body loses the ability to heal itself, the end result is death. Unfortunately, at this time, this has been the end for all those who have ever lived here on earth. No fountain of youth has been found to change that.

The biggest challenge to our health is the food supply. Mass produced food will keep us alive for a time, but will not keep us healthy because mass produced food does not give us the nutrition that is required for health. That is why we see heart disease, diabetes and cancer continuing to rise in spite of medical and governmental recommendations for diet. For example, a low fat diet is particularly harmful as it denies the body of vital nutrients for health that only saturated fat can deliver. (There are fat-soluble nutrients, such as Vitamins A, D, E and K that require saturated fat in order to be utilized by our bodies.) Whole organic milk, animal fat from grass-fed or wild caught animals and oils such as coconut and palm oil have health benefits that are vital in helping ward off degenerative diseases. (See [The Fats of Life and What You Don't Know Could Kill You](#).) Some of the smoothie recipes in this book incorporate coconut milk as a base for a reason: it is healthy.

When we take a closer look at mass produced food, we see food that is taken from plants that have problems with pests and disease and therefore require pesticides and other treatments. Plants that are healthy typically don't have problems with insects or disease. Pests generally attack plants that are not healthy. Because these plants have been grown with chemical fertilizers and not with compost, organic fertilizer and tilling under crops that will add nutrients back to the soil, the food is not as nutritious as we need it to be. Also, much of the soil the food is grown in has been stripped of its nutrients over time. This is why it is so important that we buy organically grown food as well as grass-fed and wild caught animals. Organic and natural food will help ensure that what we eat is nutritious and will put us on the road to health.

We also have an additional problem with our food supply, and that is Genetically Modified (GM, GMO) or Genetically Engineered (GE) foods that have been altered for various reasons. At this time, there is no indication on packaging in the United States to show whether or not a food is part of this group. Also, it is unknown if these foods can cause problems because not enough time has passed and not enough studies have been done to prove them safe. And we even have Frankenfish coming to our supermarkets. Have fun researching that one!

APPENDIX III - SUPPLEMENTATION

In researching nutritional information for the Superfood Series, it would appear that nutrients in food grown today are not as high as food grown 40-50 years ago. In some instances, such as the Vitamin A in apples, nutrients are about half the value of those grown years ago. What does that mean for us? That means that we need to supplement our diets with additional minerals and vitamins. Unfortunately, many available supplements are junk. They are not organic, having the carbon molecule, and can create problems by being stored by our bodies instead of being utilized.

That should prompt us to be more selective in our supplementation. Our supplements need to be liquid supplements made up of organic foods with fulvic acid. Liquid goes into the system faster and is utilized more quickly by our bodies. If made up of organic foods, these supplements will not pose problems with minerals being stored in the joints and causing arthritis or other conditions. If our food supply offered truly nutritious foods, we might not have to resort to supplementation at all.

If you question whether or not hard milled supplement tablets actually offer benefit or not, check with your local water purification system and those who handle portable bathrooms. There are tales about what these INTACT tablets do to a water supply system. Yes, our bodies lack the ability to break down some of these hard milled supplements.

These tablets are made up of rock minerals. They are not food for humans; they are food for plants. Plants have the ability to break these rock minerals down, detoxify and utilize them in a way that makes them available to us when we eat the plants and plant products. There is a very interesting article at http://www.doctorsresearch.com/articles3.html concerning the type of mineral supplements we should be taking.

Cupric Sulfate or Copper Sulfate is found in many over-the-counter supplements. The above mentioned article states:

"Copper sulfate is copper combined with sulfuric acid. It is used as a drain cleaner and to induce vomiting; it is considered as hazardous heavy metal by the City of Lubbock, Texas, that "can contaminate our water supply."

We need copper in our diets, but it needs to be organic copper. And this is just one of many minerals in supplements mentioned in this informative article.

If our food supply lacks the nutrients we need to stay healthy, it is more important than ever to make sure we eat a variety of organic foods that will supply what we need to stay as healthy as possible. Too many people are going to hospitals repeatedly with diseases and conditions they have until the only way they leave is in a body bag.

Yes, death has been the future for all mankind; but we shouldn't allow it to come sooner than it would if we took care of ourselves with good diets, stress management, sleep habits and exercise. Life is a precious gift, and we need to care for it just as we would any valuable gift. Becoming informed is the first step in caring for that life, and you have begun that process with this e-book.

APPENDIX IV – SELF MUSCLE TESTING

Muscle testing is a simple way to get information from your body in regard to various foods and other substances. Most muscle testing is done with a tester and a subject. The subject may stand and hold his arm out to his side, and the tester will try to gently pull his arm down. If food or a substance is being checked, it should be held against the abdomen as the navel is the most sensitive part of the body for this test. This allows checking for sensitivities or allergies to any substance as well.

Because the tester can sometimes influence the results, if not careful, or there is no one to do the testing, self-muscle testing can be done. Anyone can learn this simple way of getting information from his body. However, since there is no verbal response, the question is "how can I do this?" It's very simple.

Sway method - Stand up straight. Since you will be asking your body yes or no questions, you need to establish with your body that it will sway forward for yes and backward for no. Then simply ask questions with yes or no answers. Do NOT ask a question you don't want the answer to. (I.e. If you are terrified of cancer, don't ask if you have cancer. Most of us have a few cancer cells in our bodies that will never come to anything, and your body will answer 'yes' if that is the case with you.) Why does this work? It's because your body will never lie to you. Just be clear with your questions, and make sure that they can be answered with yes or no.

If the response from your body seems a little forced, relax. You may be overriding your body's response. So, then close your eyes. I guarantee that you will not be able to control the sway with your eyes closed. You body will be in complete control at that point and will be able to give you answers to your questions.

NOTE: If you have a problem with balance, stand near a wall or have someone with you when you do this type of testing.

Since this method is a little obvious in its execution, you might not want to check things in public in this manner since you might be looked upon as a 'looney tune.' There is another way to self-test that is less obvious.

Twitching finger - With this method, you establish that your little finger will twitch if the answer is yes or do nothing if the answer is no. This is very unobtrusive and can be done almost anywhere. When checking a food or other substance in public, pretend to read the label or be studying the item while holding it near your abdomen. This way you don't attract attention.

Can you ask general questions of your body?

Of course. Ever had one of those odd sensations in your body that made you uneasy? Get a little panicky about it? Just ask your body 'is this something I need to worry about?' and get your answer. If the answer is 'no,' then don't worry about it. Sometimes our bodies just make little weird adjustments that are nothing. If the answer is 'yes,' then ask more questions and find out what you need to do to take care of yourself.

What's great about self-muscle testing is that it is a non-invasive way of getting information about the state of your body whether it's your health status, need for exercise or need for sleep because you have pushed yourself to your limit and need to stop. Remember, your body will never lie to you. You can always trust the information it gives you. Keep your questions simple, and ask for more information if you need to.

NOTE: Some fainting, heart attacks or strokes may be brought on because a person panics because 'they think' they are having a heart attack or stroke. This is why you ask your body 'Is this something to worry about." If your body indicates no, then it's telling you this is nothing to worry about. Never forget that our minds are very powerful and that remaining calm in any situation will help toward positive results. That includes our health.

ABOUT THE AUTHOR

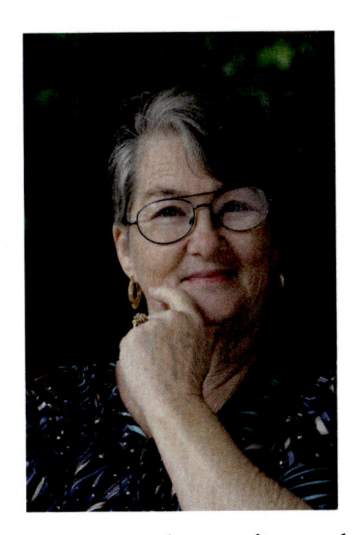

Karen Groves -- researcher, writer and teacher specializing in health issues like cancer and diabetes, natural products, superfoods, homeopathic remedies and supplements.

When asked recently why she is working on the Superfoods Series of books, Karen said, "Unfortunately, most of our food supply is contaminated with pesticides, hormones, antibiotics and other dangerous substances, not to mention Genetically Modified Organisms (GMO) foods that are invading our food supply. As a result, we need to be careful with what we put in our bodies. For better health, we should be eating organic, natural, grass fed or wild caught foods - Superfoods. So this series of Superfood books is my effort to help people make better choices for themselves and for their families."

Since 1990, Karen has worked off and on with various natural products and supplements, including products specifically formulated for cancer patients and diabetics.

As a result of her research, she has made major changes in her own diet by adding more superfoods. As a result, she is experiencing positive changes to her own health. So you might say that Karen 'practices what she preaches.'

In 1980 Karen nearly died, and that is when she was introduced to homeopathic remedies. They saved her life, and since then she has done nothing but natural medicine (homeopathic remedies, Bach flower remedies, essential oils, energy work, chiropractic treatments, massage and diet). This was quite a change for the daughter of a General Surgeon and a nurse.

COPYRIGHT NOTICE AND DISCLAIMER

Copyright © 2013 Network Performance Corporation

All Rights Reserved. No part of this publication may be reproduced in any form or by any means, including scanning, photocopying, or otherwise without prior written permission of the copyright holder.

First Printing, 2013

Printed in the United States of America

DISCLAIMER

The Publisher and Author have striven to be as accurate and complete as possible in the creation of this e-book, notwithstanding the fact that they do not warrant or represent at any time that the contents within are accurate due to the rapidly changing nature of the health/medical field.

While all attempts have been made to verify information provided in this publication, the Publisher and Author assume no responsibility for errors, omissions, or contrary interpretation of the subject matter herein. Any perceived slights of specific persons, peoples, or organizations are unintentional.

In practical advice books, like anything else in life, there are no guarantees of results. Readers are cautioned to rely on their own judgment about their individual circumstances and act accordingly.

This e-book is for information only. This e-book is not intended for use as a source of medical advice. Users are urged to seek medical advice before embarking upon or changing a course of medication or fitness program or before making extreme changes in their lifestyle. All readers are also advised to seek services of competent professionals if they are having serious medical, mental or emotional problems.